Mental Health in Historical Perspective

Series Editors
Catharine Coleborne
School of Humanities and Social Science
University of Newcastle
Callaghan, NSW, Australia

Matthew Smith
Centre for the Social History of Health and Healthcare
University of Strathclyde
Glasgow, UK

Covering all historical periods and geographical contexts, the series explores how mental illness has been understood, experienced, diagnosed, treated and contested. It will publish works that engage actively with contemporary debates related to mental health and, as such, will be of interest not only to historians, but also mental health professionals, patients and policy makers. With its focus on mental health, rather than just psychiatry, the series will endeavour to provide more patient-centred histories. Although this has long been an aim of health historians, it has not been realised, and this series aims to change that. The scope of the series is kept as broad as possible to attract good quality proposals about all aspects of the history of mental health from all periods. The series emphasises interdisciplinary approaches to the field of study, and encourages short titles, longer works, collections, and titles which stretch the boundaries of academic publishing in new ways.

More information about this series at
http://www.palgrave.com/gp/series/14806

Yolana Pringle

Psychiatry and Decolonisation in Uganda

palgrave
macmillan

Yolana Pringle
Department of Humanities
University of Roehampton
London, UK

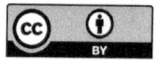

Mental Health in Historical Perspective
ISBN 978-1-137-60094-3   ISBN 978-1-137-60095-0   (eBook)
https://doi.org/10.1057/978-1-137-60095-0

Library of Congress Control Number: 2018957447

This Palgrave Macmillan imprint is published by the registered company Springer Nature Limited
The registered company address is: The Campus, 4 Crinan Street, London, N1 9XW, United Kingdom

ACKNOWLEDGEMENTS

This book, which originated in doctoral research at the University of Oxford, was made possible through the generous support of the Wellcome Trust. It is due to them that it has been published open access, and so freely available to the many scholars, medical practitioners and other interested individuals in Uganda who may not otherwise have been able to read it. Given the persistence of high barriers to research and publication in Africa, open access publishing has never been more important.

While this project was in its early stages, Sloan Mahone, my supervisor at Oxford, supported me with encouragement and critical insights, while allowing me room to pursue unexpected avenues in my own way. David Anderson, Jan-Georg Deutsch, and Pietro Corsi also provided much appreciated guidance and support. My examiners, Mark Harrison and Mike Jennings, offered helpful critiques which encouraged me to transform my research into a monograph, and suggested ways to take the project in new directions.

In Uganda, my research would not have been possible without the expert assistance of research assistants Ronald Byamukama, Robinson Kisaka, Ronald Muruya, and translators Eugene Malimba and Andrew Muhimbise. I am grateful for the guidance provided by staff at Mengo Hospital, Toro Hospital, the Church of Uganda (Rukungiri), Uganda's various district archives, the Uganda National Archives, the Albert Cook Memorial Library, Butabika Hospital, PROMETRA, the Joint Clinical Research Centre (Mbale), Makerere University, the Ministry of Health, Mental Health Uganda and the Uganda Human Rights Commission.

Seggane Musisi, Joseph Bossa, Robinah Alambuya, Kabale Benon, Eddie Nkurunungi and Stella Ndyanabangi deserve special thanks for generously sharing their warmth and time, and for encouraging me to think about my project in new and exciting ways.

I am indebted to all of the people who agreed to be interviewed and patiently answered all of my questions. Most respondents have been anonymised in order to protect their privacy, but this by no means diminishes their importance. Moreover, I thank Allen German, Jim Wood, John Orley, Wilson Acuda and Diane Zeller for responding enthusiastically to my requests for information and clarification, and supplying me with some invaluable unpublished materials.

An earlier version of Chapter 4 was published as Y. Pringle, 'Investigating "Mass Hysteria" in Early Postcolonial Uganda: Benjamin H. Kagwa, East African Psychiatry, and the Gisu', *Journal of the History of Medicine and Allied Sciences* 70(1) (2015), pp. 105–136. I thank Oxford University Press for permission to reproduce some of this material here.

In addition to support from the Wellcome Trust, I have benefited from funding from Jesus College, Oxford, and the British Institute in Eastern Africa. The bulk of the work to transform my research into this monograph was done as a result of the freedom afforded by a Mellon-Newton Interdisciplinary Postdoctoral Research Fellowship at the Centre for Research in the Arts, Social Sciences and Humanities (CRASSH) at the University of Cambridge. The University of Cambridge's Returning Carers Scheme, which allowed me to follow up on new research leads in Uganda, deserves special mention not only for its role in shaping the later chapters of the monograph, but for its importance (particularly for early career women) in aiding the transition back to academia after a career break.

During the research and writing of this monograph, more people than I am able to acknowledge here have provided support and much-needed perspective. Special thanks must nevertheless go to Charlotte Cross, Nicki Kindersley, Dan Branch, Roberta Bivins, Harriet Palfreyman, Michelle Sikes, Pat Stys, Kathleen Vongsathorn, Andrea Grant, Lynsey Shaw and Belinda Clark. The series editors Matt Smith and Cathy Coleborne, as well as Oliver Dyer and Molly Beck at Palgrave Macmillan, have expertly guided me through the publication process, while the anonymous reviewers have provided critical insights and encouraged me to do more with my sources. New colleagues at the University of Roehampton have encouraged the final push to get this monograph out.

My mother, Mariette, who is more inspirational than she knows, has always encouraged me to pursue education. Her love and support cannot be thanked enough.

Finally, apart from being my intellectual sounding board and best friend, my husband, Tim, has been a constantly supporting voice. I look forward to spending more time with him, with Zoe, and with Nicholas, who has become far too used to me hiding away to 'work on the computer'.

Contents

Abbreviations

ACMM	Albert Cook Memorial Library, Makerere University
AMO	African Medical Officer
BOD	Bodleian Library, University of Oxford
CEHURD	Centre for Health, Human Rights and Development
CMS	Church Missionary Society
DC	District Commissioner
DMS	Director of Medical Services
DMSS	Director of Medical and Sanitary Services
DPM	Diploma in Psychological Medicine
DSM	Diagnostic and Statistical Manual of Mental Disorders
ECT	Electroconvulsive Therapy
JDA	Jinja District Archives
KDA	Kabale District Archives
MDA	Mbale District Archives
MHAC	Mental Health Advisory Committee
MMU	Mountains of the Moon University, Fort Portal
MO	Medical Officer
NAMH	National Association for Mental Health
PCO	Psychiatric Clinical Officer
PSW	Psychiatric Social Worker
SDA	Soroti District Archives
TNA	The National Archives, Kew, UK
UMOHA	Uganda Ministry of Health Archives
UMOHL	Uganda Ministry of Health Library
UNA	Uganda National Archives
WFMH	World Federation for Mental Health

WHO   World Health Organization
WHOA   World Health Organization Archives, Geneva
WHOL   World Health Organization Library, Geneva

CHAPTER 1

Introduction

In April 1969, twenty-five psychiatrists from nine African countries, the UK and the USA met at Makerere University College in Kampala, Uganda, to discuss the organisation of mental health services in Africa. Among them were several 'giants' of African psychiatry, including Tolani Asuni, then of Aro Hospital, Nigeria, Taha A. Baasher, then of Khartoum North psychiatric outpatient clinic, Sudan, C. C. Adomakoh, of Accra Mental Hospital, Ghana, and Stephen B. Bosa, of Butabika Hospital, Uganda. Over three days, the participants considered the roles of psychiatrists in developing countries, the size and scope of psychiatric institutions, problems of stigma and outdated legislation, alternative forms of care, the use of auxiliary health workers and postgraduate training. They attended the opening of an exhibition of paintings of mental patients organised by the Uganda National Association for Mental Health (NAMH) and took advantage of the opportunity to socialise and exchange ideas—an opportunity that was highly welcome for those psychiatrists who worked single-handedly in their own countries.[1]

The discussions made it clear that there was no one vision for the future of mental health care in Africa. While some participants argued that existing mental hospitals, inherited from colonial rule, needed to form the basis of a 'modern' mental health care system on the grounds of economic and administrative efficiency, others were more cautious, highlighting cases of 'social catastrophe' or stigmatisation following admission. A few went so far as to demand the closure of mental hospitals altogether,

© The Author(s) 2019
Y. Pringle, *Psychiatry and Decolonisation in Uganda*,
Mental Health in Historical Perspective,
https://doi.org/10.1057/978-1-137-60095-0_1

stressing that hospitalisation was 'anti-therapeutic' and pointing to moves to close large psychiatric institutions in Europe and the USA. Discussions on alternative forms of care, meanwhile, highlighted a wide variety of experiments in progress, including music therapy, village settlements and rural psychiatric outpatient clinics, as well as mixed opinions on group therapy and the value of traditional healers.[2] Even the role of the psychiatrist in a developing country was up for debate. In the dual contexts of decolonisation and nation building, the central question for participants was whether they should remain primarily in custodial and curative roles. Did they have a duty to contribute their expertise to issues of social planning and national development? On this question, one group maintained that psychiatrists needed to focus on the curative aspects of the profession, particularly as knowledge about the causes of mental illness and the significance of rapid social changes in developing countries was limited. The other group, by contrast, did not want to be limited to a single role. They saw their education, intelligence and expertise as raising a moral imperative to act. The psychiatrist, they stressed, 'must be prepared to take on many mantles, and must be prepared to offer advice in those areas of social planning which were likely to influence the mental health and happiness of people'.[3] These views, according to G. Allen German, Professor of Psychiatry at Makerere, reflected differences in human personality, the variety of which could be accommodated in mental health services in Europe and the USA: 'In developing countries, however, where personnel are few, it may be that one man will have to adopt different roles, and this is one of the problems of working in a developing society which has to be accepted'.[4]

The meeting in Kampala was just one of several regional and international meetings on the practical problems of mental health care delivery in developing countries held between the late 1960s and the mid-1970s. They reflected the increasingly transnational character of psychiatry in the mid-twentieth century and belied any simplistic North–South or Western/non-Western transmission of knowledge or expertise. Psychiatrists gathered in Hong Kong in 1968, Chile in 1969, and Singapore and Cairo in 1970, with the participation of psychiatrists from developing countries made possible through the financial support of international organisations who were starting to look beyond Europe to problems of mental health worldwide.[5] The Kampala meeting had been sponsored by the Commonwealth Foundation and the World Federation for Mental Health (WFMH), but they were not the only organisations involved. In 1970, an inter-regional seminar on the organisation of psychiatric services in the Soviet Union (USSR) was facilitated by the United Nations Development Programme (UNDP) and the World Health Organization (WHO), bringing together nineteen psychiatrists and public health officers from fourteen developing countries, including India, Mexico, Japan, Uganda and Tanzania. Over two weeks, the participants shared experiences from their own countries and studied how the USSR had established a network of psychiatric services in urban and rural areas, and their relationship with general health, social welfare and educational services.[6] In January 1971, moreover, the Indian Psychiatric Association and the WFMH organised a workshop bringing together psychiatrists and clinical psychologists from across India to review the shortcomings of existing mental health services and draw up recommendations for future development. These recommendations included more investment in mental health training for general practitioners and auxiliary health workers, the revision of the 1912 Lunacy Act, the expansion of outpatient care centres and the appointment of a full-time advisor on mental health at the level of central government.[7]

Concern about the organisation of mental health services in developing countries was, in many ways, a logical extension of research conducted since the 1950s that was challenging many of the earlier held assumptions of psychiatrists under colonial rule. Work within both psychiatric epidemiology and transcultural psychiatry, a sub-discipline that was concerned with the presentation and management of mental illness across different cultures, was suggesting that mental disorders once regarded as comparatively rare in developing countries, such as depression, were in fact as common as elsewhere in the world. This research was also challenging fears that urbanisation and education would lead to increased rates of mental disorder, highlighting instead the ways in which such social changes might make communities less willing or able to care for the mentally ill, as well as the inadequacy of the mental health system bequeathed by the colonial powers.[8] As a series of review articles on psychiatry in Africa, South America and South-East Asia commissioned by *The British Journal of Psychiatry* in 1972–1973 made clear, the expansion of mental health services in developing countries was a necessary part of social and economic development—pressure on existing services would only increase in the coming years.[9]

At a more fundamental level, however, concern about the organisation of mental health services reflected what might be termed as a 'crisis of legitimacy' among psychiatrists at the end of empire. Under colonial rule, psychiatry had in many territories been limited to a single mental hospital and a specialist European medical officer who may or may not have had training in psychiatric or psychological medicine. It was under-funded by colonial governments, of low status within the colonial medical hierarchy, and had little to offer its patients therapeutically. As many psychiatrists in developing countries were well aware, psychiatry still lingered on the edge of a much broader therapeutic landscape. While transcultural psychiatry, pursued by many newly trained indigenous-born psychiatrists, had from the 1950s offered renewed hope of a more culturally sensitive and patient-centred approach to psychiatry, there were few easy answers as to how psychiatrists might bridge what was a huge social and cultural gulf between psychiatry and its patients. During the period of decolonisation, then, psychiatrists in developing countries had to contend not only with an ongoing lack of resources and specialist personnel, but with their lack of social, cultural and professional legitimacy. Expressing his frustration at the problems facing psychiatry, particularly in Africa, Ayo Binitie, of the Nervous Diseases Clinic, Benin City, Nigeria, noted in 1974 that one of the most important difficulties facing mental health care planners was the 'communication gap'—'between the public and the psychiatrist, between the psychiatrist and the health administrator, and between psychiatrists and governments. In some countries there are no psychiatrists so that there is not even the beginning of dialogue'.[10]

It was against this backdrop of discussion and debate among psychiatrists that the WHO sought to provide strategic direction in the 1970s, notably through an inter-regional seminar on the organisation of mental health services in Addis Ababa, Ethiopia, in late 1973, and an Expert Committee on the Organisation of Mental Health Care Services in Developing Countries in Geneva in October 1974.[11] While the papers presented at these meetings highlighted the wide variety of new approaches and methods being tried by psychiatrists in developing countries, the final *Report* of the Expert Committee, published in 1975, presented a coherent agenda for future mental health policy and research. Stressing that low levels of specialist personnel and funding required innovative approaches to mental health care in developing countries, the *Report* advocated that responsibility for mental health be shared between psychiatrists, general health workers and a range of community agencies. Psychiatrists would need to be trained in teaching and supervising, and then supported to implement new programmes, taking into account the needs and resources of their individual countries. This strategy of integrating mental health into primary (general) health care would go on to form the basis of WHO policy on mental health, itself in alignment with the focus on primary health care and development at the lowest possible cost that would soon be established at the Alma-Ata Conference in 1978.

This book locates Uganda and Uganda's psychiatrists within this reimagining of psychiatry and mental health care at the end of empire. I examine the challenges facing a new generation of psychiatrists as they took over responsibility for psychiatry, and explore the ways psychiatric practices were oriented towards and responded to shifting political and economic contingencies, periods of instability and tension, and a broader context of transnational and international exchange. I argue that the distinctiveness of psychiatry in the early postcolonial era is that of a culture of experimentation and creativity, something that was, fundamentally, a response to a new contextually sensitive politics. In Uganda, while the institutions of psychiatry remained largely unchanged during the decades of decolonisation, psychiatrists aimed to refigure the relationship between psychiatry and the mentally ill in light of the needs and priorities of development and nation building, as well as an awareness of the professional, economic and cultural constraints on psychiatric practice. Their activities represented an attempt to extend the reach of psychiatry in novel ways at a time when colonial institutions needed to demonstrate their relevance, and when globally, the authority of psychiatry was increasingly coming under attack, not least through deinstitutionalisation. Yet while the approaches trialled in Uganda contributed to the development of international policy on the organisation of mental health services in developing countries, there remained a large gap between intentions and practices within Uganda. Psychiatric practices were contested and negotiated, and the power of psychiatry limited, not least by patients themselves. Through an in-depth historical study of Uganda, I contend that the reorientation of psychiatry during the decades of decolonisation was no straightforward process. Nor was it one that was entirely successful.

Psychiatry and Decolonisation in Africa

The period of decolonisation saw the human sciences being mobilised for empire on an unprecedented scale. The establishment of the Colonial Social Science Research Council (CSSRC) in 1944, following the 1940 Colonial Welfare and Development Act, channelled the first significant amounts of funding for the social sciences into Africa. This included the establishment of the East African Institute for Social Research (EAISR) at Makerere in 1948, under the guidance of Audrey Richards, and which was host to research on patterns of social change, the effects of urbanisation, attitudes to Europeans, 'traditional' law, land tenure systems and acculturation (or culture contact).[12] Psychological concepts and expertise were also at the heart of psychological warfare, or the battle for 'Hearts and Minds', in counter-insurgency operations in Malaya, Cyprus, Kenya, Algeria and Southern Rhodesia.[13] Psychiatrist and philosopher Frantz Fanon spoke of the effects of physical and psychological violence on suspected nationalist sympathisers in Algeria's 'brainwashing centers', while psychiatrist J. C. Carothers was commissioned by the Kenya Government to study the causes and nature of the Mau Mau rebellion (1952–1960).[14] Carothers framed Mau Mau as a pathology stemming from the inability of Africans to cope with 'the transition between the old ways and the new'.[15] While he noted the importance of economic and historical grievances, 'both real and imagined', Mau Mau was the inevitable result of 'an anxious conflictual situation in people who, from contact with the alien culture, had lost the supportive and constraining influences of their own culture, yet had not lost their "magic" modes of thinking'.[16] Mau Mau oaths, existing 'in all the depravity that is imaginable', therefore had a profound psychological effect on initiates, and required all the tactics of the government's 'Screening Teams' to break their hold.[17]

The application of psychological and psychiatric knowledge to the problems of empire was not new. Since the early twentieth century, ethnopsychiatry, a field of study concerned with the psychology and behaviour of non-Western peoples, had developed a powerful language through which to understand the native psyche and to usefully articulate the problems facing colonial administrators.[18] While ethnopsychiatry had its intellectual roots in the comparative psychiatry of Emil Kraepelin and the writings on primitive mentalities by Sigmund Freud, it largely comprised a loose group of individuals with varying levels of medical training, including the esteemed psychiatrist Antoine Porot, as well as Wulf Sachs, J. B. F. Laubscher, Carothers, and the teacher and self-taught psychoanalyst J. F. Ritchie.[19] Between the 1920s and the 1950s, when ethnopsychiatry in colonial Africa was at its height, much of their writing revolved around the problems of acculturation, or culture contact, a facet which bound the field to anthropology, and presupposed that psychiatric knowledge could be applied to political issues. Within the 'East African School of Psychiatry and Psychology', as it became known, H. L. Gordon, Visiting Physician to Mathari Mental Hospital, Kenya, 1930–1937, stressed how his experience at Mathari had shown him that mental illness in Africans was primarily organic in origin, and that the peculiarities of African psychopathology could be explained by fundamental differences between Africans and Europeans in brain size and growth. Carothers, who followed Gordon at Mathari, emphasised the importance of cultural, as opposed to biological difference (though he by no means saw these as discrete categories). He argued that a number of mental disorders frequently seen in Europe, such as depression and the neuroses, were completely absent in East Africa.[20] More overt forms of 'mental derangement', by contrast, were increasingly common, as 'detribalisation'—something that encompassed such diverse aspects as 'Christianization, secular education, working relationships with non-African employers, relationships with Government officials and with shop-keepers (the latter mostly Indian), life in townships, and the introduction of syphilis and alcoholic spirits and other drugs'—took hold.[21] The failure of African cultures to incorporate the traits of individual control, abstract thought and personal responsibility, it was theorised, meant that 'westernisation' and 'detribalisation' were particularly dangerous for Africans and required the immediate extension of 'social protection and control'.[22]

Acknowledging the ways in which anthropologists, psychologists and psychiatrists informed colonial policies, or provided theories that were attractive to colonial officials and settlers, is not to state that the human sciences were unproblematic tools of empire.[23] Many of these 'experts' negotiated multiple and often ambiguous roles within colonial structures and institutions, and their professional and intellectual ambitions frequently bore little resemblance to their daily practice. This was particularly the case within psychiatry, where theories about acculturation and detribalisation were rarely reflected in diagnostic categories or treatment regimes. Ethnopsychiatric theories tended to focus on the collective, rather than the individual; they were warnings that African societies were, as a whole, becoming psychologically unstable. It is noteworthy that only a small number of those under the grip of Mau Mau's collective 'madness', for example, were regarded as clinically insane. While individuals who challenged colonial rule could face charges of mental illness, particularly if they exhibited violent behaviour, in most cases, psychiatry was simply not an effective tool of social or political control. Firstly, the processes of confinement were laborious, involving examination by two registered medical practitioners who had to agree on a diagnosis, which then had to be accepted by a magistrate. Secondly, suggestions of mental illness conflicted with desires to see 'troublemakers' prosecuted under law and set as an example to others.[24]

What an examination of psychiatry at the end of empire forces us to confront is that colonial psychiatry, more generally, was not a unified force. Colonial governments and military leaders may have been enthralled by the possibilities offered by psychological knowledge, but the methodologies, aims and assumptions of researchers varied considerably. Even as Carothers' WHO-sponsored monograph, *The African Mind in Health and Disease,* hit the shelves in 1952, the racial and cultural determinism it espoused was already under dispute. Criticisms came from a range of disciplines. It involved Americans, Europeans and a new generation of indigenous-born and Western-trained psychiatrists.[25] Nigerian psychiatrist Thomas Adeoye Lambo described the work of a number of ethnopsychiatrists, including Carothers, as being: 'At their worst...glorified pseudo scientific novels or anecdotes with a subtle racial bias; at their best...abridged encyclopedias of misleading information and ingenious systems of working hypotheses, useful for the guidance of research, but containing so many obvious gaps and inconsistencies, giving rise to so many unanswerable questions, that they can no longer be seriously presented as valid observations of scientific merit'.[26] G. I. Tewfik, moreover, Specialist Alienist at Mulago Mental Hospital, Uganda, likened such psychiatric literature to racial prejudice towards Jews in Europe, stressing that 'Criticisms of one race by another have been shown to be nearly always fallacious. Man is a very poor judge of his fellows'.[27]

In the context of decolonisation, research that questioned the assumptions of ethnopsychiatry about racial and cultural difference—whether implicitly or explicitly—represented a strand of a broader project in which psychiatrists were making professional and political claims to equality. As Matthew Heaton has convincingly argued, Nigerian psychiatrists were acutely aware of the political significance of their research, contributing to the deracialisation of psychiatric theories not just in Africa, but globally, through participation in major international collaborative research projects and conferences.[28] Lambo's central role in the Cornell-Aro Mental Health Research Project, for example, not only led to a methodology for effective cross-cultural comparison of major psychiatric disorders (in this case between the Yoruba and Canadian communities), but also helped to undermine assumptions about the relationship between race, culture and mental illness.[29] Similar claims can be made for psychiatrists elsewhere in Africa, including Uganda, where psychiatrists were also involved in developing new methodologies, including clinical interviews, field surveys, hospital and government records, and psychological questionnaires. In doing so, psychiatrists in Africa actively shaped the nascent fields of transcultural psychiatry and psychiatric epidemiology, and embarked on a process of decolonising some of the more insidious aspects of colonial psychiatry. Yet psychiatric theories represented only one legacy of colonial rule. The decolonisation of psychiatry needed to include psychiatric practices and a reconfiguration of the dynamics of power, too. Here, change was much more uneven.

While histories of colonial psychiatry have provided us with a picture of psychiatric practices and discourses that are remarkably consistent across geographical contexts, there is no one history of psychiatry and decolonisation.[30] 'Africanisation', a political process consisting of policies aimed at increasing the number of Africans in the colonial administration through training and promotion, was patchy at best within psychiatry. By the late 1960s, Uganda, Nigeria and Senegal represented the few countries in Africa (excluding South Africa) with formal programmes for the training of psychiatrists and psychiatric nurses, and consequently could boast of considerably more African psychiatrists within psychiatric institutions. Psychiatrists in newly independent countries also often had very different ideas about how psychiatry might best be developed. In a statement on Senegal, but which could apply to Africa more generally, Alice Bullard has noted that with independence, 'Colonial psychiatry transformed into a diverse range of practices, ranging from collaborations with traditional healing to biomedical, pharmaceutical-based psychiatry'.[31] Such innovations included the introduction of the *accompagnant* at the Fann Psychiatric Clinic, Dakar, in 1972, comprising a family member or close friend who stayed with a patient during their hospitalisation, and which claimed 'its genesis in "traditional" African ways of life'.[32] In Nigeria, moreover, Heaton has shown that the political context of decolonisation allowed psychiatrists not only to argue for the deracialisation of psychiatric theories, but also to experiment with community-based psychiatry and collaborations with traditional healers. The most famous of these new schemes was Lambo's Aro Village project, founded in 1954, and consisting of a day hospital attached to four villages. Patients, who were accompanied by at least one relative, were boarded out in the villages where, in addition to the physical therapies received at the hospital, they could be employed on nearby farms and participate in daily village life.[33] Such experiments were exceptional, however; they were often expensive and made many psychiatrists—expatriate and African alike—uneasy about the implications for the status of psychiatry as a 'modern' science.[34] Most newly independent governments, moreover, were scarcely more interested in investing in or experimenting with mental health care than their predecessors. This was most visible in the institutions themselves, as Richard Keller has commented for the Maghreb, where well into the postcolonial era they 'represented the only real resource for managing mental illness'.[35]

Shifting historiographical periodisation away from the artificial divide of colonial/postcolonial to decolonisation, which for a history of psychiatry should span the first moves towards Africanisation following the Second World War, to the political crises of many African states during the 1970s and 1980s, allows for deep analysis of continuities and divergences in psychiatric practices, not only in relation to colonial rule, but also between countries in Africa. As I show in this book, the capacity of psychiatrists to reform psychiatric practices, to contribute to international debates and to provide care for patients was tied to the changing social, political and economic contexts in which they worked. Some of the continuities, such as the ongoing concentration of resources and personnel in a single mental hospital, need to be seen as necessities, as psychiatrists struggled to convince newly independent governments to commit the vast sums required to reorganise mental health services. Many of the divergences, meanwhile, can be usefully framed as responses and contributions to the evolving needs and priorities of development, nation building, modernisation and manpower, as well as the ability to access funding and to travel. Yet all, ultimately, need to be linked to shifting periods of political stability, upheaval and crisis, which challenged the ability of psychiatry to successfully decolonise.

Psychiatry as a Transnational and Global Phenomenon

Since the mid-twentieth century, psychiatry has constituted an increasingly transnational and global body of knowledge and practices, which no history of psychiatry and decolonisation can ignore. This transnationalism was not in itself new to psychiatry. The development of psychiatry in colonial settings, as historians of psychiatry and empire have demonstrated, was not simply the result of a uni-directional flow of ideas from the metropole, but involved psychiatrists, particularly in South Asia, engaging in discussions about concepts and approaches both within and beyond empire.[36] In Europe and the USA during the 1920s, moreover, the rise of international health organisations and a broader spirit of collaboration saw discussion of mental health move beyond predominantly national confines to address comparative approaches to institutional care, law, social welfare and training.[37] The International Committee on Mental Hygiene (ICMH) was founded in 1919 to advocate for mental hospital reform and to encourage mental health in 'normal' populations, with numerous national branches. The ICMH's 1930 International Congress, held in Washington DC, brought together over 3000 participants from twenty-two countries, predominantly European in origin, but including the USSR, India, Japan, Siam, Venezuela and the Union of South Africa.[38] It was not until after the Second World War, however, that patterns of transnational communication and exchange changed significantly in a process that was inextricably linked with a project of modernity and what Marijke Gijswijt-Hofstra and Harry Oosterhuis have called 'a more general process of psychologisation - a change of mentality combining growing individualisation, internationalisation, and self-guidance, related to changing social manners and relationships'.[39] It is from the mid-twentieth century that ideas and practices within psychiatry started to be increasingly similar in different geographical and cultural contexts. This move towards universalism was cemented by the development of universal diagnostic criteria, as exemplified in the WHO's International Classification of Diseases 9 (ICD-9) in 1975, as well as the American Psychiatric Association's Diagnostic and Statistical Manual of Mental Disorders III (DSM-III) in 1980, yet is one that has belied a single explanation. Historiographically, it has been tied to the rise and power of international health organisations, the pursuit of progress and modernity within psychiatry, and the need of psychiatry to reform and unify in the face of various crises since the 1950s.[40] This book adds an additional perspective—that of shared challenges facing psychiatrists in developing countries, which stimulated debate on new ways to organise mental health services, and which directly fed into the development of WHO policy.

Two international health organisations occupied central positions within the increasingly transnational and international field of psychiatry and mental health: the WHO and the WFMH. The WHO was established in 1948 as a specialised agency of the United Nations (UN) and whose mission, according to Javed Siddiqi, was infused with notions of spillover theory, in which international cooperation in public health might 'spillover' into the political arena by promoting peace and security around the world.[41] The creation of the WHO's Mental Health Unit shortly after the founding of the WHO reflected this broader aim, coinciding with optimism within policy circles about the ability of psychiatric and psychological expertise to assist in post-war reconstruction and rehabilitation efforts.[42] Notions of a broader purpose were also present in the aims of the WFMH, founded in 1948 under the leadership of John Rawlings Rees, a British military psychiatrist, with the assistance of George Brock Chisholm, a Canadian psychiatrist and first Director-General of the WHO. In its founding document, 'Mental Health and World Citizenship', the WFMH declared that 'the ultimate goal of mental health is to help [people] live with their fellows in one world'.[43] It understood 'world citizenship' as a form of 'common humanity' in which individual and cultural differences needed to be respected. Both the WFMH and the WHO foregrounded the importance of mental health in broader public health efforts, taking as their goal the need to understand the psychosocial as well as biological causes of mental disorder, a field of study that would become known as 'social psychiatry'.[44]

The WHO and the WFMH spurred an international mental health field by facilitating the formation of a series of loose networks of psychiatrists and related professionals who exchanged research and practical experiences via international meetings and conferences. The WHO's Expert Committee on Mental Health met on a yearly basis to discuss such themes as the training of psychiatrists, psychosomatic disorders and the role of general practitioners in mental health care, as well as to suggest recommendations for member states.[45] Psychiatrists from around the world were also in attendance at the International Congresses of the WFMH and the World Congresses of the World Psychiatric Association (WPA), founded in 1961, and which included a Transcultural Psychiatry Section. Yet manpower, along with political and economic dynamics within newly formed nation states, often restricted the ability of psychiatrists from developing countries to take part in the internationalism that increasingly characterised psychiatry during the decades of decolonisation. For those in developing countries, participation in international mental health more commonly took the form of what Sunil Amrith has called the 'administrative pilgrimages' or 'journeys by a coterie of experts' that saw regional and inter-country exchanges.[46] The WHO and the WFMH were important actors here, not only as a source of financial support, but because they were free from political links with former colonial powers, making their input politically acceptable.[47] Yet, as Nitsan Chorev has made clear, the WHO, far from being a neutral actor, was itself an agent of international health, with officials at the WHO Secretariat, Geneva, actively seeking to shape policy.[48] Nor was internationalism free from regional interests or international politics. Political and economic connections between Kenya, Tanganyika and Uganda, forged under British colonial rule and cemented with the East African Community in 1967, were reflected in ongoing close links between psychiatrists in East Africa. Former British and French colonies also found that language difficulties restricted interactions within networks of psychiatry, despite the Association of Psychiatrists in Africa, founded in 1969, making a concerted effort to involve both English- and French-speaking nations. Psychiatrists also deliberately avoided holding meetings in apartheid South Africa, and were to be found travelling to non-aligned India and the USSR, but not to countries geopolitically situated in the US sphere of influence, such as South America.

The power of international health organisations in the latter half of the twentieth century has been their ability to structure and mobilise knowledge: to classify and organise information, to fix meanings by establishing parameters of action and to diffuse universal norms and standards.[49] Within the WHO, the first Chief of the Mental Health Unit, Ronald Hargreaves, envisaged large-scale cross-cultural research projects, with the ultimate aim of understanding the global landscape of mental disorders.[50] Hargreaves and his successors pursued this through the development of rigorous methodology for large epidemiological surveys, drawing on research already being undertaken by psychiatrists in Scandinavia as well as other European and American contexts. The result was the launch of the WHO's International Pilot Study of Schizophrenia in 1966, which tested the cultural applicability of translated versions of a diagnostic tool for schizophrenia, the Present State Examination, across nine research centres in different countries.[51] The study, which published its first results in 1973, concluded that while symptoms, or the 'cultural colouring' of schizophrenia, might vary in different cultural settings, it was possible to develop criteria for its diagnosis cross-culturally.[52] Such findings were central to the development of a universal diagnostic system for psychiatric illnesses, as established in ICD-9. This trend towards universalism within the WHO was not limited to diagnostic categories, however. From the 1970s, the WHO also sought to develop a methodology for collecting information on and assessing the effectiveness of mental health services around the world. Following the 1974 Expert Committee on the Organisation of Mental Health Services in Developing Countries, the Collaborative Study on Strategies for Extending Mental Health Care aimed to assess different techniques for community-based mental health care, with the aim of both refining its own guidelines on the organisation of mental health care and providing evidence through which they could convince member states to integrate mental health into national health care plans.[53] Such attempts at collecting standardised data were largely unsuccessful, however. Instead, the WHO continued to base policy on the collective knowledge and shared experiences of psychiatrists engaged in the reorganisation of mental health care in their own countries. This approach confirms for Africa, and indeed developing countries more generally, what Steve Sturdy, Richard Freeman and Jennifer Smith-Merry have shown for Europe—that the role of the WHO in setting policy on mental health services has been one of creating opportunities for the emergence of an 'epistemic community', in which 'context-sensitive knowledge' rather than 'standardised forms of data' has been key.[54]

Participation in the epistemic communities making up the field of international mental health has represented a key expression of modernity, not least for the psychiatrists who have been able to make claims to international, if not global citizenship. The pursuit of progress and modernity has pervaded psychiatry throughout the twentieth century, in developing countries as much as in Europe and the USA.[55] And it has taken multiple forms—it has involved psychiatrists keeping up to date with research published in international journals, the deliberate use of English as a dominant language of communication, the formation of new research collaborations and the adoption of the latest treatments and technologies—forms that have not been without their own politics.[56] In developing countries, the pursuit of modernity among psychiatrists was inextricably linked to the politics of decolonisation and development. In Nigeria, as Matthew Heaton has made clear, many psychiatrists were closely engaged in a project of modernity, yet they 'did not simply buy into the idea that Western ideas could be universally applied to bring about the development of the emerging Third World'. Instead, they sought to adapt and rework psychiatric ideas and practices so they could be regarded as both universal and culturally specific.[57] In Argentina, moreover, according to Andrew Lakoff, psychiatrists felt an intense pressure to pursue a global professional identity, yet found themselves fiercely opposed to the biological model of mental illness espoused by the DSM, itself in conflict with their own psychoanalytic model and 'unresolved project of social modernity'.[58] The pursuit of 'modernity' was certainly not synonymous with 'westernisation'. Nor did it mean that psychiatric theories and practices were adopted without contestation or adaptation. Rather, it provoked tensions between 'modernity' and 'westernisation' that psychiatrists in developing countries struggled to resolve.

It is no coincidence that the trend towards universalism within psychiatry globally occurred at a time when psychiatry faced a series of challenges to its own authority over mental illness. In Europe and the USA, psychiatry's hegemony over mental illness was increasingly challenged from the 1950s by deinstitutionalisation, attempts to extend patients' legal rights, the expansion of new counselling and psychotherapy services, and the intellectual critiques of the antipsychiatry movement.[59] In the USA, the crisis facing psychiatry created the conditions in which psychiatry moved from an environmental and behavioural model of mental illness to that of the biological, symptom-based classificatory scheme represented by DSM-III. This 'revolution' in psychiatry, according to Rick Mayes and Allan V. Horwitz, was couched in the language of 'objectivity, truth, and reason'.[60] It allowed psychiatrists to measure mental illness in a 'scientific' manner, helping to 'silence the critics of the previous system, who claimed that mental illnesses could not be defined in any objective way', and thus provided legitimacy to a profession under attack.[61] There was no comparable antipsychiatry movement in developing countries. Yet, as I argue in this book, psychiatrists in Uganda, and indeed more generally in Africa, were acutely aware of their lack of social, cultural and professional legitimacy. While most were only one of a handful of psychiatric professionals working within their own countries, these shared challenges proved a unifying force. They not only spurred experimentation in local settings, but stimulated debate on mental health services at transnational and international levels. Running through these discussions were questions about the role psychiatrists in developing countries should have, not only in relation to their patients, but to other health workers, legal professionals, and community agencies. In Uganda, as I show in this book, efforts to mobilise other professionals in support of psychiatry constituted an attempt to extend the reach of psychiatry at a time when psychiatry was facing increasing constraints on its power. While attempts to refigure the place of psychiatry within other institutions and services were not entirely successful within Uganda, the experiences of psychiatrists nevertheless proved influential in wider discussions on mental health services in developing countries, representing one of the first attempts to articulate mental health in primary care.

Recognising psychiatry as a transnational and global phenomenon is to acknowledge that late colonial and postcolonial histories of psychiatry cannot be told as isolated national stories, and certainly not through the lens of colony (or former colony) and metropole. Yet we must be careful not to erase or overlook the social, cultural and professional contexts in which psychiatrists worked. Indeed, these have been central not only in shaping the priorities and aims of psychiatrists, but in determining the ability to travel and participate in debates. As the Uganda case makes clear, despite a period of intense activity in the late 1960s and early 1970s, in the longer term, psychiatrists in Africa faced barriers to participation that resulted in disproportionately few contributions to research and policy both within their own countries and at transnational and international levels. These imbalances of power were reinforced in many contexts in the 1980s and 1990s by structural adjustment policies, which undermined national health care systems, civil wars and internal conflict, and the emergence of an international humanitarian aid industry that increasingly turned its attention to the mental health and psychological consequences of war and violence. Humanitarian psychiatry, and new techniques of psychological counselling that developed alongside it, not only universalised a particular type of suffering body, but privileged westernised notions of distress and trauma.[62] Since the 1990s, moreover, the global mental health movement, which aims 'to improve services for people living with mental health problems and psychosocial disabilities worldwide, especially in low- and middle-income countries where effective services are often scarce', has become a dominant force in the global psychiatric landscape. It has been challenged as 'colonial medicine come full circle, a modern-day version of Kipling's 'White Man's Burden', full of good intentions, but also a form of anthropologically uninformed cultural imperialism'.[63] What this book aims to do is to provide a historical investigation into the conditions in which these developments have been deemed possible, even necessary.

PSYCHIATRY IN UGANDA

Uganda may at first seem an unusual choice for a history of psychiatry and decolonisation. Next to Kenya, home to the infamous East African School of Psychiatry and Psychology, there was little to distinguish psychiatry in Uganda under colonial rule. Like most other countries in Africa, Uganda had for most of the colonial period only one mental hospital: Hoima, Mulago and then Butabika. Reflecting the low priority accorded to psychiatry, provision for the mentally ill also came long after the formal establishment of Uganda as a British Protectorate in 1894. Hoima Prison, in western Uganda, was officially designated as a Lunatic Asylum only in 1921, with minimal attempt made to offer patients anything more than custodial care. This was followed in 1935 by a new, purpose-built mental hospital on a site near Mulago Hospital, Kampala, in central Uganda, which promised to treat mental illness by psychiatric means for the first time. By the late 1940s, overcrowding had reached such an extent that plans were made to build a new mental hospital at Butabika, seven miles outside of Kampala. The first patients were transferred to Butabika Hospital in 1955, and in 1964, Mulago Mental Hospital was closed for good. It was only at Independence in 1962 that the first attempts were made at outpatient and non-custodial care: first through a mental health clinic at Mulago Hospital and then in 1964 through the designation of 'Ward 16' for the treatment of a small selection of mental patients.[64] In the organisation and day-to-day running of these mental hospitals, there was also little that made Uganda unique. The general underdevelopment and neglect, poor sanitary conditions, overcrowding, the importation of psychiatric practices from Europe (including the English nineteenth-century 'moral management' regime), the copying of lunacy legislation from other colonies, and the reproduction of colonial hierarchies of race, gender and class in the organisation and management of inmates are all common themes in the history of psychiatry and empire. So too is the fragile hold of psychiatry by the end of colonial rule, with psychiatry remaining, perhaps more than any other medical discipline introduced under colonialism, on the periphery of a much broader therapeutic landscape.

Psychiatry in colonial Uganda was neglected and underdeveloped as a field. Nevertheless, during the years of decolonisation, psychiatrists and other medical practitioners saw themselves as uniquely placed to address questions about the future of psychiatry in Africa.

This stemmed not from an existing tradition of psychiatric research and practice, but from the commitment to training and research at Makerere Medical School, first opened at Mulago Hospital in 1923.[65] When the school was opened, there was only one other medical school for Africans on the continent (in Dakar, Senegal), and the training of Africans in medicine quickly became one of the defining features of Uganda's Colonial Medical Service. While European medical officers did not always regard their African colleagues as equals, they nevertheless believed that their training programmes set Uganda apart as more liberal than other colonies, and in particular from Kenya.[66] During the 1940s and 1950s, when medical practitioners from across Eastern and Southern Africa raised concerns about the ability of Europeans to understand their African patients, it was Makerere that responded. By the late 1960s, Uganda was one of the few countries in Africa that could train psychiatrists and psychiatric nurses in country, foregoing the need to send them overseas. Following the opening of a Department of Psychiatry in 1966, moreover, a new group of Ugandan and expatriate psychiatrists established Africa's first mental health association, the NAMH, introduced programmes for training and delegating responsibility to a range of health care workers, and developed psychiatric training and research to a point where it could no longer be ignored by health and legal professionals. Uganda gained a reputation both within Africa and the WHO as a place of innovation and reform. 'Mental health services in Uganda', as the WHO African Mental Health Action Group acknowledged in 1987, were 'once the best in the region'.[67]

The drive to reorganise mental health services stemmed from the challenges facing psychiatrists, particularly in reaching their patients. This theme of distance between psychiatry and those it seeks to help runs through the book. The idea that Africans had natural cultural insight into mental illness, which could be harnessed for clinical practice and research, fed into the first calls for the training of Ugandans in psychiatry. Initial optimism had faded by the 1960s, however, as it became clear that people were scarcely more likely to turn to psychiatry when facing mental illness. The newly independent Uganda Government, moreover, proved little more interested in listening to the ideas of Ugandan psychiatrists than had their colonial predecessors.

Following the opening of the Department of Psychiatry, the need to extend the reach of psychiatry both within and beyond the walls of the mental hospital became central to justifying new experiments and training programmes. In the contexts of development and nation building, these efforts to reform mental health services were framed as the 'psychiatry of poverty', in which the limited ability of governments to invest in psychiatric services and manpower not only distinguished psychiatry in Africa from that in Western contexts but required new ways of thinking about the use of non-specialists in mental health care. Uganda was not unique in facing these challenges—discussions about how best to organise mental health care, and the implications this might have for psychiatrists, would dominate the agendas of regional and international conferences over the next decade. This collective experience would play a key role in bringing psychiatrists together on a regional basis, as well as coming to shape the direction of international mental health policy. Notably, the experiences of psychiatrists in experimenting with mental health care within their own countries, particularly through training and delegation, would provide the basis for the WHO's policy on mental health in primary care. Yet the innovations in psychiatry during the late 1960s and early 1970s had minimal impact on the reach of psychiatry in Uganda. The power of psychiatry was repeatedly challenged, not only through the practical difficulties of effecting change with few resources and personnel, but by patients, who continued to assert their agency as they navigated psychiatric services in which they were given no official say. Yet the limits on psychiatry were most prominently brought to the fore in the 1970s and 1980s, when Uganda faced political and economic insecurity, firstly under the rule of Idi Amin, who took power following a coup in January 1971, and then in the violence of the successive regimes that followed.[68] Psychiatry was not only brought to the brink of collapse, but it was not regarded as an appropriate agent to deal with distress associated with conflict or violence. Since the 1980s, the limited role of psychiatry has only been exacerbated by the influx of humanitarian and non-governmental organisations concerned with trauma and Post-Traumatic Stress Disorder, and the ongoing marginalisation of the mentally ill within health and social welfare systems. Psychiatry might have 'Africanised', but it has by no means decolonised.

NOTES

1. *Mental Health Services in the Developing World: Reports on Workshops on Mental Health, Edinburgh (1968) and Kampala (1969)*, Commonwealth Foundation Occasional Paper IV (Hove, 1969); World Health Organization Archives (WHOA) NIE-HMD-002 Jkt 1 (Medical School, University of Ibadan); A. Boroffka, 'The Delivery of Mental Health Care', n.d.
2. *Mental Health Services in the Developing World*, pp. 38–41.
3. Ibid., p. 33.
4. Ibid.
5. G. M. Carstairs, 'Psychiatric Problems of Developing Countries', *The British Journal of Psychiatry* 123(574) (1973), pp. 271–277; Organizacion Panamericana de la Salud, *Grupo de Trabajo Sobre La Administración de Servicios Psiquiátricos y de Salud Mental, Vina Del Mar, Chile, 14–19 de Abril de 1969* (Washington, DC, 1970).
6. *The Work of WHO 1970: Annual Report of the Director-General to the World Health Assembly and to the United Nations* (Geneva, 1971), pp. 81, 269.
7. World Health Organization Library (WHOL) SEA/Ment./19 Annex 7, 'Recommendations of the International Workshop on Priorities in Mental Health Care (held in Madurai, from 21 to 22 January 1971, under the auspices of the World Federation for Mental Health)', n.d.
8. The history and implications of this research are addressed in Chapters 5 and 6 of this book, as well as: J. Bains, 'Race, Culture and Psychiatry: A History of Transcultural Psychiatry', *History of Psychiatry* 16 (2005), pp. 139–154; M. M. Heaton, *Black Skin, White Coats: Nigerian Psychiatrists, Decolonization, and the Globalization of Psychiatry* (Ohio, 2013).
9. J. S. Neki, 'Psychiatry in South-East Asia', *The British Journal of Psychiatry* 123(574) (1973), pp. 257–269; C. A. Leon, 'Psychiatry in Latin America', *The British Journal of Psychiatry* 121(561) (1972), pp. 121–136; and G. A. German, 'Aspects of Clinical Psychiatry in Sub-Saharan Africa', *The British Journal of Psychiatry* 121(564) (1972), pp. 461–479.
10. World Health Organization Library (WHOL) OMH/EC/74.7, A. Binitie, 'Mental Health Services in Developing Countries with Special Reference to Africa', Paper Presented to the Expert Committee on Organization of Mental Health Services in Developing Countries, Geneva, 22–28 October 1974, p. 3.
11. T. A. Baasher et al., eds., 'Mental Health Services in Developing Countries', Papers Presented at a WHO Seminar on the Organization of Mental Health Services, Addis Ababa, 27 November to 4 December 1973 (Geneva, 1975); World Health Organization, *Organization of Mental Health Services in Developing Countries, Sixteenth Report of the WHO Expert Committee on Mental Health* (Geneva, 1975).

12. D. Mills, 'British Anthropology at the End of Empire: The Rise and Fall of the Colonial Social Science Research Council, 1944–1962', *Revue d'Histoire des Sciences Humaines* 6(1) (2002), pp. 161–188.
13. E. Lindstrum, *Ruling Minds: Psychology in the British Empire* (Cambridge, MA, 2016), Ch. 5.
14. F. Fanon, *The Wretched of the Earth*, trans. R. Philcox (New York, 1963), pp. 213–216.
15. J. C. Carothers, *The Psychology of Mau Mau* (Nairobi, 1955).
16. Ibid., p. 15.
17. Ibid., pp. 15–16.
18. S. Mahone, 'East African Psychiatry and the Practical Problems of Empire', in S. Mahone and M. Vaughan, eds., *Psychiatry and Empire* (Basingstoke, 2007); J. McCulloch, *Colonial Psychiatry and 'The African Mind'* (Cambridge, 1995).
19. W. G. Jilek, 'Emil Kraepelin and Comparative Sociocultural Psychiatry', *European Archives of Psychiatry and Clinical Neuroscience* 245(4–5) (1995), pp. 231–238; J. McCulloch, *Black Peril, White Virtue: Sexual Crime in Southern Rhodesia, 1902–1935* (Bloomington, IN, 2000); and H. Pols, 'Psychological Knowledge in a Colonial Context: Theories on the Nature of the "Native Mind" in the Former Dutch East Indies', *History of Psychology* 10(2) (2007), pp. 111–131.
20. On the East African School, see especially: G. C. Beuschel, 'Shutting Africans Away: Lunacy, Race and Social Order in Colonial Kenya, 1910–1963' (Unpublished PhD thesis, University of London, 2001); S. Mahone, 'The Psychology of the Tropics: Conceptions of Tropical Danger and Lunacy in British East Africa' (Unpublished DPhil thesis, University of Oxford, 2004); and McCulloch, *Colonial Psychiatry*.
21. J. C. Carothers, 'A Study of Mental Derangement in Africans, and an Attempt to Explain Its Peculiarities, More Especially in Relation to the African Attitude to Life', *East African Medical Journal* 25(5) (1948), pp. 153–154.
22. J. C. Carothers, 'A Study of Mental Derangement in Africans, and an Attempt to Explain Its Peculiarities, More Especially in Relation to the African Attitude to Life', *East African Medical Journal* 25(5) (1948), pp. 217–218; M. Vaughan, *Curing Their Ills: Colonial Power and African Illness* (Cambridge, 1991), Ch. 5.
23. This point is also made by Lindstrum in *Ruling Minds*.
24. S. Mahone, 'The Psychology of Rebellion: Colonial Medical Responses to Dissent in British East Africa', *Journal of African History* 47(2) (2006), pp. 241–258.

25. WHOA M4/445/13. See, for example, M. J. Herskovits, 'The African Mind in Health and Disease: A Study in Ethnopsychiatry by J. C. Carothers', Man 54 (1954), p. 30.
26. T. A. Lambo, 'The Role of Cultural Factors in Paranoid Psychosis Among the Yoruba Tribe', The British Journal of Psychiatry 101(423) (1955), p. 241.
27. G. I. Tewfik, 'Mulago Hospital Clinical Staff Meeting April 26, 1958: The African Mind Fact or Myth?' East African Medical Journal 35(8) (1958), p. 512.
28. Heaton, Black Skin, White Coats.
29. Ibid., Ch. 2.
30. The now substantial body of literature on colonial psychiatry includes: W. Ernst, Mad Tales from the Raj: Colonial Psychiatry in South Asia, 1800–58 (London, 2010); L. Jackson, Surfacing Up: Psychiatry and Social Order in Colonial Zimbabwe, 1908–1968 (Ithaca and London, 2005); R. C. Keller, Colonial Madness: Psychiatry in French North Africa (Chicago, 2007); J. Mills, Madness, Cannabis and Colonialism: The 'Native Only' Lunatic Asylums of British India, 1857 to 1900 (Basingstoke, 2000); J. Parle, States of Mind: Searching for Mental Health in Natal and Zululand, 1868–1918 (Scottsville, 2007); J. Sadowsky, Imperial Bedlam: Institutions of Madness in Colonial Southwest Nigeria (Berkeley and Los Angeles, 1999); M. Vaughan, 'Idioms of Madness: Zomba Lunatic Asylum, Nyasaland, in the Colonial Period', Journal of Southern African Studies 9(2) (1983), pp. 218–238; and S. Mahone and M. Vaughan, eds., Psychiatry and Empire (Basingstoke, 2007).
31. A. Bullard, 'Imperial Networks and Postcolonial Independence: The Transition from Colonial to Transcultural Psychiatry', in S. Mahone and M. Vaughan, eds., Psychiatry and Empire (Basingstoke, 2007), p. 197.
32. K. Kilroy-Marac, 'Of Shifting Economies and Making Ends Meet: The Changing Role of the Accompagnant at the Fann Psychiatric Clinic in Dakar, Senegal', Culture, Medicine and Psychiatry 38(3) (2014), pp. 427–447.
33. Heaton, Black Skin, White Coats, Chs. 2, 5.
34. Heaton has also made this point for Nigeria.
35. Keller, Colonial Madness, p. 196.
36. W. Ernst, Colonialism and Transnational Psychiatry: The Development of an Indian Mental Hospital in British India, c. 1925–1940 (London, 2013); W. Ernst and T. Mueller, eds., Transnational Psychiatries: Social and Cultural Histories of Psychiatry in Comparative Perspective c. 1800–2000 (Newcastle, 2010); and S. Kapila, 'The "Godless" Freud and His Indian Friends: An Indian Agenda for Psychoanalysis', in Mahone and Vaughan, eds., Psychiatry and Empire.

37. P. Weindling, ed., *International Health Organisations and Movements, 1918–1939* (Cambridge, 1995).
38. M. Thomson, 'Mental Hygiene as an International Movement', in Weindling, ed., *International Health Organisations and Movements, 1918–1939.*
39. J. C. Burnham, 'Transnational History of Medicine After 1950: Framing and Interrogation from Psychiatric Journals', *Medical History* 55(1) (2011), pp. 3–26; M. Gijswijt-Hofstra and H. Oosterhuis, 'Introduction: Comparing National Cultures of Psychiatry', in M. Gijswijt-Hofstra et al., eds., *Psychiatric Cultures Compared: Psychiatry and Mental Health Care in the Twentieth Century: Comparisons and Approaches* (Amsterdam, 2005), p. 15.
40. M. Gijswijt-Hofstra et al., eds., *Psychiatric Cultures Compared: Psychiatry and Mental Health Care in the Twentieth Century: Comparisons and Approaches* (Amsterdam, 2005); Heaton, *Black Skin, White Coats*; N. Henckes, 'Narratives of Change and Reform Processes: Global and Local Transactions in French Psychiatric Hospital Reform After the Second World War', *Social Science & Medicine* 68(3) (2009), pp. 511–518; A. Lakoff, *Pharmaceutical Reason: Knowledge and Value in Global Psychiatry* (Cambridge, 2006); and R. Mayes and A. V. Horwitz, 'DSM-III and the Revolution in the Classification of Mental Illness', *Journal of the History of the Behavioral Sciences* 41(3) (2005), pp. 249–267.
41. J. Siddiqi, *World Health and World Politics: The World Health Organization and the UN System* (London, 1995).
42. On the early work of the WHO's Mental Health Unit, see World Health Organization, *WHO and Mental Health 1949–1961* (Geneva, 1962).
43. As cited in E. B. Brody, 'The World Federation for Mental Health: Its Origins and Contemporary Relevance to WHO and WPA Policies', *World Psychiatry* 3(1) (2004), pp. 54–55.
44. H. Y.-J. Wu, 'World Citizenship and the Emergence of the Social Psychiatry Project of the World Health Organization, 1948–c. 1965', *History of Psychiatry* 26(2) (2015), pp. 166–181.
45. See, for example, World Health Organization, *Psychosomatic Disorders: Thirteenth Report of the Expert Committee on Mental Health* (Geneva, 1964); World Health Organization, *The Role of Public Health Officers and General Practitioners in Mental Health Care: Eleventh Report of the Expert Committee on Mental Health* (Geneva, 1962); and World Health Organization, *Training of Psychiatrists: Twelfth Report of the Expert Committee on Mental Health* (Geneva, 1963).
46. S. S. Amrith, *Decolonizing International Health: India and Southeast Asia, 1930–65* (Basingstoke, 2006), p. 14.

47. J. Pearson-Patel, 'French Colonialism and the Battle Against the WHO Regional Office for Africa', *Hygiea Internationalis* 13(1) (2016), pp. 65–80.
48. N. Chorev, *The World Health Organization Between North and South* (Ithaca, 2012).
49. M. N. Barnett and M. Finnemore, 'The Politics, Power, and Pathologies of International Organizations', *International Organization* 53(4) (1999), pp. 710–715.
50. H. Y.-J. Wu, 'From Racialization to World Citizenship: The Transnationality of Taiwan and the Early Psychiatric Epidemiological Studies of the World Health Organization', *East Asian Science, Technology and Society* 10(2) (2016), pp. 183–205; Wu, 'World Citizenship'.
51. J. L. Cox, 'Aspects of Transcultural Psychiatry', *The British Journal of Psychiatry* 130(3) (1977), p. 218.
52. World Health Organization, *Report of the International Pilot Study of Schizophrenia* (Geneva, 1973).
53. World Health Organization, *Mental Health Care in Developing Countries: A Critical Appraisal of Research Findings: Report of a WHO Study Group* (Geneva, 1984); N. Sartorius and T. W. Harding, 'The WHO Collaborative Study on Strategies for Extending Mental Health Care, I: The Genesis of the Study', *American Journal of Psychiatry* 140 (1984), pp. 1470–1473.
54. S. Sturdy, R. Freeman, and J. Smith-Merry, 'Making Knowledge for International Policy: WHO Europe and Mental Health Policy, 1970–2008', *Social History of Medicine* 26(3) (2013), pp. 532–554.
55. See, for example, the chapters in: Gijswijt-Hofstra et al., eds., *Psychiatric Cultures Compared*.
56. Burnham, 'Transnational History of Medicine After 1950'.
57. Heaton, *Black Skin, White Coats*, p. 5.
58. Lakoff, *Pharmaceutical Reason*, p. 44.
59. G. N. Grob, 'The Attack of Psychiatric Legitimacy in the 1960s: Rhetoric and Reality', *Journal of the History of the Behavioral Sciences* 47(4) (2011), pp. 398–416; D. V. Kritsotaki, V. Long, and M. Smith eds., *Deinstitutionalisation and After: Post-War Psychiatry in the Western World* (Basingstoke, 2016).
60. Mayes and Horwitz, 'DSM-III and the Revolution', p. 250.
61. Mayes and Horwitz, 'DSM-III and the Revolution', p. 251.
62. D. Fassin and R. Rechtman, *The Empire of Trauma: An Inquiry into the Condition of Victimhood* (Princeton, 2009); B. Taithe, 'The Cradle of the New Humanitarian System? International Work and European Volunteers at the Cambodian Border Camps, 1979–1993', *Contemporary European History* 25(2) (2016), pp. 335–358; and M. Vaughan, 'Changing the

Subject? Psychological Counseling in Eastern Africa', *Public Culture* 28(3) (2016), pp. 499–517.

63. R. Whitley, 'Global Mental Health: Concepts, Conflicts and Controversies', *Epidemiology and Psychiatric Sciences* 24(4) (2015), p. 289. See also: S. Cooper, 'Global Mental Health and Its Critics: Moving Beyond the Impasse', *Critical Public Health* 26(4) (2016), pp. 355–358; G. Miller, 'Is the Agenda for Global Mental Health a Form of Cultural Imperialism?', *Medical Humanities* (Published online 13 March 2014), pp. 1–4; C. Mills and S. Fernando, 'Globalising Mental Health or Pathologising the Global South? Mapping the Ethics, Theory and Practice of Global Mental Health', *Disability and the Global South* 1(2) (2014), pp. 188–202; V. Patel and M. Prince, 'Global Mental Health: A New Global Health Field Comes of Age', *JAMA* 303(19) (2010), pp. 1976–1977; and D. Summerfield, 'Afterword: Against "Global Mental Health"', *Transcultural Psychiatry* 49(3–4) (2012), pp. 519–530.

64. Mahone, 'The Psychology of Rebellion'; J. F. Wood, 'A Half Century of Growth in Ugandan Psychiatry', *Uganda Atlas of Disease Distribution* (Kampala, 1968).

65. The school was referred to as Mulago Medical School from 1927 and Makerere Medical School from 1939.

66. On medical education, see C. Campbell, *Race and Empire: Eugenics in Colonial Kenya* (Manchester, 2007); W. D. Foster, 'Makerere Medical School: 50th Anniversary', *British Medical Journal*, 3(5932) (1974), p. 675; J. Iliffe, *East African Doctors: A History of the Modern Profession* (Kampala, 2002); M. Lyons, 'The Power to Heal: African Medical Auxiliaries in Colonial Belgian Congo and Uganda', in D. Engels and S. Marks, eds., *Contesting Colonial Hegemony: State and Society in Africa and India* (London, 1994); A. M. Odonga, *The First Fifty Years of Makerere Medical School and the Foundation of Scientific Medical Education in East Africa* (Kampala, 1989); and C. Sicherman, *Becoming an African University: Makerere, 1922–2000* (Trenton, 2005), Ch. 8.

67. WHOL MNH/POL/87.3, *African Mental Health Action Group, Tenth Meeting, Geneva, 8 May 1987*, p. 8.

68. On Uganda's social and political history since 1962, see especially: S. R. Karugire, *A Political History of Uganda* (Kampala, 2010); A. B. K. Kasozi, *The Social Origins of Violence in Uganda, 1964–1985* (Montreal, 1994); P. Mutibwa, *The Buganda Factor in Uganda Politics* (Kampala, 2008); and R. Reid, *A History of Modern Uganda* (Cambridge, 2017).

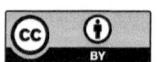

CHAPTER 2

A Place on Mulago Hill

The memoirs and other writings of missionaries, travellers and physicians in colonial Uganda are full of accounts of the powerful impression western medicine made on the 'native' mind. Cures for syphilis by injections of Salvarsan '606', or of procedures to remove cataracts, were credited with helping to convince Africans of the benefits Europeans could bestow, whether in the form of Christianity or 'civilisation'. As Church Missionary Society (CMS) doctor Albert Ruskin Cook recalled on his earliest surgeries, which were performed in front of audiences: 'Anaesthetics were at first a great marvel; on seeing no sign of pain while extensive wounds were inflicted and large tumours etc. removed with the necessary loss of blood, some thought we had killed the patient. On the effects of the anaesthetic passing off and the suffering exhibiting signs of life, some credited us with raising the patient from the dead'.[1] While such self-congratulatory and often patronising accounts were common among medical missionaries and physicians, few made such bold claims about mental illness. This was due in part to the invisibility of mental cases, more frequently cared for at home, leading some Europeans to question whether mental disorder existed as a distinct disease category in Africa, separate from organic disease. But it was also linked to an awareness that western medicine had little to offer by way of therapeutic hope, particularly as explanatory frameworks for understanding and treating mental illness were so different. It was a rare boast for Philip Hutton, at Mulago Hospital from 1937 to 1961, to recall how:

© The Author(s) 2019
Y. Pringle, *Psychiatry and Decolonisation in Uganda*,
Mental Health in Historical Perspective,
https://doi.org/10.1057/978-1-137-60095-0_2

One of the views held by local Africans was that there were two kinds of illness:- Those which could be cured by injections and those which were only amenable to 'native medicine' i.e. the practise of witchdoctors. Those would have appeared to be of a psychological or psychiatric nature. On one occasion having 'cured' a case of hysterical blindness with suggestion assisted by pentothal I was constantly being stopped and congratulated by members of staff for having cured an 'African' disease with an injection.[2]

The history of psychiatry in colonial Uganda reflects this marginal nature of psychiatry within broader systems of healing, as well as within the colonial medical hierarchy. Psychiatry existed in Uganda not because it was particularly useful or effective, but because it was regarded by the colonial administration as a logical method of dealing with madness in a civilised society. Charles Baty, Superintendent of Mulago Mental Hospital, expressed this sentiment in a lecture to mental hospital attendants in the early 1940s. He described how 'Many years ago there were no Mental Hospitals in Africa and mad people just went walking about and sometimes died, and sometimes they killed people and set fire to houses and stole and did damage to other peoples [sic.] property'.[3] 'Sometimes', he added, 'they were caught and chained up in a little house and kept there until they died or got better'.[4] Yet these conditions were 'very troublesome both for the people who look after mad people and for the mad people themselves, so Uganda like all other African countries came to have a Mental Hospital because lunatics are less troublesome and the country is much safer when lunatics are kept in a place by themselves where they are properly looked after and where they will have the best chance to recover'.[5] For Baty, the establishment of institutions for the confinement of the mentally ill was a sign of progress and of the benevolence of British rule. It was a narrative that presupposed a unity and purpose to psychiatry that privileged the power of individual psychiatrists and ignored the multiple ways psychiatry was used and contested by patients and their families.

In colonial Uganda, 'psychiatry' consisted for the most part of a fragmented group of prison warders, hospital attendants, and African and European doctors who declared authority over the mentally ill. In the archival record, it is their voices that predominate, with the identities and experiences of patients obscured—reduced to statistical tables or anonymised objects of treatment. With patient case notes from the early days of Mulago Mental Hospital having been lost or destroyed, we now know more about the brands of electroconvulsive therapy (ECT) machines used at Mulago Mental Hospital, and the numbers who underwent treatment, than we do about the lives of those who were confined. But the rare glimpses we do have of patients—in surviving court records, annual reports and administrative correspondence—point to their creativity and resourcefulness, whether through challenges to the legal system, refusing to maintain order, or by resorting to hunger strikes. Such instances, often little more than archival echoes, remind us that colonial psychiatry was not an all-encompassing force. Not only was there no 'great confinement' in Africa to match that of nineteenth-century Europe, as Megan Vaughan has shown us, but as a system of practices which sought control over bodies and minds, the power of colonial psychiatry was limited.[6]

The broader story told in this chapter is, in many ways, an unexceptional one within colonial Africa. Between 1894 and 1962, the dates of formal colonial rule in Uganda, provision for the mentally ill evolved from the occasional and haphazard isolation of troublesome lunatics to an established (if often flawed) system of certification, confinement and repatriation. The perception that the mentally ill would be best treated at Kampala, coupled with a series of scandals, forced the colonial government's Medical Department to acknowledge responsibility for the mentally ill. If there was no overarching scheme for psychiatry, however, it was not because it was isolated from wider medical, social or political trends. One of the most distinctive features of western medicine in early colonial Uganda, for example, was the strong medical missionary presence. In the period before 1940, medical practice was marked by a high level of collaboration between mission doctors and the Colonial Medical Service, with a number of CMS doctors negotiating dual roles as missionaries and colonial medical officers.[7] An even greater number participated in and managed government health campaigns or were engaged unofficially by the administration in an advisory capacity. When the colonial government sought advice on the development of psychiatry from the 1920s, they turned to medical missionaries, notably the CMS doctor Albert Cook, for advice.[8] In the longer term, however, it was the colonial government's interest in medical training that would have significant implications for psychiatry. As seen through the development of a medical school at Mulago Hospital from 1923 (referred to as Mulago Medical School from 1927 and Makerere Medical School from 1939), the training of Africans in medicine soon came to dominate colonial medicine in Uganda and, for some doctors, was a point of pride.[9] While European doctors did not always regard their African colleagues as equals, they nevertheless believed that their training programmes set Uganda apart as more 'liberal' than other colonies, and in particular from Kenya.[10] The ways that African doctors occupied complicated and often ambiguous positions within the power structures of psychiatry is explored in Chapter 3. Most important for the purposes of this chapter, however, was the nature of colonial rule in Uganda. Unlike Kenya, Uganda's neighbour and oft-looked to point of comparison by colonial officials, Uganda did not have a large European population. While the opinions of Europeans, particularly those living in the main area of European residence, Kampala, were often considered, the colonial government did not have to accommodate the demands of a powerful settler community. This was significant for psychiatry because it meant that the development of what we might deem to be institutions of 'social control', and associated legislation and policy, were less urgent. Hoima Asylum was formally opened in 1921, almost thirty years after the establishment of the Uganda Protectorate in 1894, and significantly later than Kenya's Mathari Asylum, which opened on the outskirts of the Nairobi Municipal Area in 1909.[11] Also reflective of the small European population was the minimal provision made for European patients, even after the opening of Mulago Mental Hospital in 1935. These features fed into the predominantly reactive nature of psychiatry in colonial Uganda: changes to policy, or to buildings and accommodation, frequently occurred following a perceived problem created either by a European or African patient.

This chapter, which focuses on psychiatry under colonial rule, is included within this book because it sets up the institutions and practices that were inherited by a newly independent Uganda in 1962. The low priority accorded to psychiatry, expressed through minimal financial resources and few specialist personnel, was cemented during this period, and proved difficult for psychiatrists to change after Independence. It was also during this period that the most enduring stereotypes and assumptions about psychiatry were formed and hardened: the language of 'lunacy' and 'persons of unsound mind', the notion of psychiatry as a last resort for only the most 'difficult' or 'violent' cases, and of the mental hospital as an alienating place, where communication was difficult, if not impossible. Yet at the same time, I aim through this chapter to highlight the marginal nature of psychiatry—a recurring theme throughout the book. Those suffering from mental distress, and their families, continued to make decisions about care and treatment that were often unconnected to government or psychiatric policy.

FROM HOIMA TO MULAGO

In 1901, brothers and fellow CMS doctors Albert and Jack Cook notified the colonial government and the medical community in Britain of concerns over the growing number of sleeping sickness cases arriving at the CMS Mengo Hospital, Kampala, sparking international interest in a disease that was to devastate local communities on the shores of Lake Victoria.[12] The role assumed by the mission doctors at Mengo Hospital, and the manner in which they informed and advised the Colonial Medical Service, was to shape medical practice in Uganda, including that related to mental illness, for the next thirty years. The epidemic, which killed an estimated 250,000 people, prompted the forcible depopulation by the government of areas infested with tsetse flies, the establishment of government sleeping sickness camps, and the rapid development of a Colonial Medical Service aimed at understanding and limiting the disease.[13] Given this context, it is unsurprising that early discussion of mental pathology in Uganda was linked to sleeping sickness. Preoccupied by the volume of sleeping sickness patients who exhibited signs of mental degeneration, other types of mental illness were rendered almost invisible. As the author of an early draft of the colonial *Blue Book* of 1908–1909 commented: 'Mania and dementia apart from [in] sleeping sickness are so uncommon that their presence leads to the suspicion of the existence of that disease'.[14]

Special provision for late-stage sleeping sickness patients within government camps pre-dated the establishment of a lunatic asylum by over twenty years. These patients frequently exhibited violent or unpredictable behaviour, and as such their separation was deemed necessary for camp security. Following a visit to the camp at Kyetume, just over four miles from Mukono, central Uganda, in 1909, Albert Cook described how 'One compound was set apart for the treatment of maniacal cases, and here were half a dozen or so who had their legs shackled together to prevent them doing harm to themselves or others. They seemed far from melancholy'.[15] Writing for a similar audience, J. C. M. Baker, wife of a Medical and Sanitary Officer and camp administrator, recounted how one night: 'New sounds bore into my brain, ears are awake and strained instantly. Cries far away, quick, high-pitched, lapping over each other like ripples—the cries of alarmed natives'.[16] While in its late stages, sleeping sickness can result in mania, instances of 'difficult' behaviour, aggression and attempts to escape by detainees were consistently labelled as insane or 'irrational'. In the written record at least, little reflexivity or agency was allowed, despite widespread recognition that sleeping sickness camps were looked on with 'dread and aversion'. When, in 1909, a large number of sleeping sickness cases 'gave considerable trouble and frequently attempted to set fire to their quarters', the Governor of Uganda, Henry Hesketh Bell, explained away what was most likely a riot by declaring the perpetrators to be 'demented', and arguing for further medical care.[17]

The sleeping sickness epidemic demonstrated to the authorities in Uganda that diseased Africans could be dangerous and unpredictable, but it had little impact on policies towards the mentally ill. When the first Lunacy Ordinance was passed in 1906, it was done to provide a legal basis through which to handle the few European cases of insanity, rather than African patients.[18] Before this point, the High Court of Uganda had lacked the power to deal with 'several cases of lunacy among white men', including a Police Sergeant diagnosed with general paralysis of the insane (GPI), who needed to be sent back to England 'as soon as possible in order that he may be placed under suitable restraint'.[19] The ordinance allowed the court to certify cases of insanity following the receipt of two medical certificates, to take possession of and manage property in Uganda, and to make arrangements for custody and care. One of the first Europeans to come under the new ordinance—a senior customs official with the colonial administration—was 'apparently suffering from the effects of some severe shock to his mental system' rendering him 'incapable of managing himself or his affairs'.[20] As Uganda lacked 'special provision' for 'persons of unsound mind', his invaliding to England was deemed essential, and he remained under the constant supervision of one Medical Officer (MO) while the colonial government fought over who should be responsible for the costs.[21] Europeans found insane in Uganda would continue to be removed as long as the colonial government or relatives agreed to pay the costs, either for a journey back to England, or to mental hospitals in Kenya or South Africa.[22] While the colonial government made provision for Europeans within Hoima Lunatic Asylum from 1921 and then at Mulago Mental Hospital from 1935, the inadequacy of the accommodation and lack of staff meant it was considered undesirable to admit Europeans for anything longer than a short period prior to their transfer.

Provision for mentally ill Africans who came to the attention of the colonial administration, primarily through the police, was similarly lacking. Neither the prisons nor the medical service wanted to assume responsibility, seeking ways to avoid the financial and logistical burden as far as possible. By 1913, Hoima Prison, in western Uganda, had developed a reputation as a dumping ground for leper and insane prisoners.[23] This, according to the Inspector General of Police and Prisons, was unacceptable: 'To intern the demented, the diseased, and those in full possession of their health and senses in one and the same building when that building is lacking the means of complete segregation, is a measure so diametrically opposed to the precepts both of Prison and Medical Administration'.[24] Numbers were small—there were eleven certified lunatics at Hoima in 1914–1915—but there was minimal medical supervision (the nearest medical officer lived thirty-seven miles away) and inmates who were found to be 'difficult' were 'hand cuffed (or leg cuffed or both) to the bars of the doors of their cells'.[25] It was not until 1921 that the housing of the mentally ill with prisoners was deemed by the government to be unacceptable on logistical and moral, if not medical grounds. In that year, Hoima was gazetted as a Lunatic Asylum, and in 1923, the general prison population was removed, leaving the 'ordinary' and criminal lunatics in the remaining buildings.[26]

The repurposing of Hoima Prison as a Lunatic Asylum came just as the Colonial Medical Service in Uganda started to be reorganised. In line with growing cotton and coffee trade and a rapidly expanding European population, the colonial administration found themselves faced with the need to increase the size and scope of medical provision at minimal cost.[27] While one way of achieving this was by harnessing missionary manpower through formal contractual arrangements, the pursuit of 'efficiency' primarily meant centralisation.[28] Declaring the specialist anti-venereal disease clinics that had been at the heart of both government and missionary medical and morality campaigns since the early twentieth-century as exorbitantly expensive, moves were made to combine general and specialist medical work in all areas.[29] Here, the CMS Mengo Hospital, which by the mid-1920s had developed into a complex of medical units under one administrative head, served as the ideal model.[30] As part of their moves to reorganise medical services, the colonial administration put forward a plan for a new purpose-built mental hospital in or near Kampala, at the time a growing centre of European residence. This would reduce the amount of travelling required by patients, as well as administrative and medical staff, and allow for easier access to medical facilities. It would avoid, it was hoped, a repeat of a scandal in 1920 that saw two 'harmless lunatics' die after being forced to travel over 140 miles (a distance that took on average two full days by motor-van) from Hoima to Kampala for observation and certification.[31] Seeking the advice of physicians in Kampala— Albert Cook among them—G. J. Keane, Director of Medical and Sanitary Services (DMSS), suggested two potential sites. The first was at Luzira, a few miles outside of Kampala. While its relative remoteness from European residence would avoid the 'annoyance of the possible noise made by maniacal cases', it was far from other medical facilities in Kampala and close to Luzira Prison.[32] This, Keane warned, may serve to perpetuate 'the association of ideas which has arisen between crime and lunacy which it is desirable to end'.[33] The other site, near Mulago Hospital, would by contrast allow 'regular treatment of cases and daily and nightly supervision by medical staff', in addition to savings affected by the sharing of kitchen, laundry and cleaning services.[34]

Discussions about the proposed mental hospital forced the colonial government to consider the management of the mentally ill in more than just logistical and financial terms for the first time. Consideration now had to be given to perceptions of mental patients as noisy, unmanageable and potentially dangerous. This was not linked to large numbers of certified lunatics—at the beginning of 1930, Hoima Lunatic Asylum had only 61 inmates (38 male and 23 female, all African).[35] Nor was there any public outburst of alarm over the presence of 'raving maniacs' on the streets, as was seen in Nigeria,[36] if reports of madmen stealing 'a roll of toilet paper from the lavatory', 'placing large stones and sticks across the road', or entering the bedroom of a European woman did occasionally appear in English-language newspapers.[37] Rather, it stemmed from Hoima's origins as a prison, combined with official policy which, due to limited accommodation, urged that only the most 'urgent' or violent patients be recommended for admission.[38] All other cases, as DMSS J. Hope Reford stressed in 1926, 'should be handed to their relatives'.[39]

Mulago Mental Hospital was opened in 1935 on Mulago hill, previously home to numerous Kings of Buganda, beyond the edges of European settlement, and host to a growing number of government medical institutions, including Mulago Hospital and its medical school, opened in 1923. Mulago marked a compromise between those who wanted the mentally ill to receive specialist medical care and a broader sentiment that a 'screaming raving lunatic should never be exposed to the public'.[40] Indeed, it was hailed as a most progressive way of dealing with the mad. Modelled on the late nineteenth-century English asylum, it had, on opening, ward accommodation for 72 male and 24 female patients, as well as sixteen single isolation cells. It was set in a grass compound, with day shelters and a small garden, all surrounded by a fence. The Luganda newspaper *Gambuze* informed readers in a piece of propaganda that the Uganda Government was building a hospital for *eddwaliro ly'abalalu* (mad people) on Mulago hill 'so the staff of Mulago can look after them'. It called on readers not to take their relatives anywhere else, for 'this will be where the mentally ill will be taken for treatment'.[41] *Matalisi* similarly described how the colonial government intended to 'bring learned foreigners' to work at this new specialist hospital. The English-language *Uganda Herald*, meanwhile, proclaimed that 'Like all modern institutions of its kind, the 'padded cell' is done away with as it is understood that really obstreperous patients are treated with drugs'. But, it was careful to add, the wards would be painted with 'special paint' to prevent escapes, all windows would be fastened from the outside, and 'the buildings...so erected that it is not anticipated any noise will be heard by the patients in Mulago [General] hospital'.[42] Such perceptions about noise would prove difficult to overcome. As an anecdote among Mulago Hospital staff in the 1970s relayed, when the site for the mental hospital buildings was chosen, administrators sent 'a large group of hospital employees and their wives on a noisy progress from the General Hospital, and, when their din could no longer be heard...the site for the new hospital was marked!'[43]

CASES FOR ADMISSION

The decision to open a new mental hospital at Mulago marked an intention to treat mental illness by 'modern' psychiatric means for the first time. It did not represent a shift in the types of patients deemed suitable for admission, however. Until 1956, admissions to the mental hospital were involuntary, dependent on reports made by chiefs, the police and two medical practitioners, and were determined by a system that continued to prioritise 'unmanageable' and violent cases.[44] Numbers also grew rapidly throughout the colonial period, with the total number of annual admissions rising from 24 in 1935 to 652 (including 26 read-missions) in 1956.[45] The explanations for this were subject to debate, with some suggesting that rising numbers was evidence of the inability of Africans living in urban settings to cope with the demands of 'civi-lisation'.[46] Writing in 1951, Uganda's first Specialist Alienist, George Campbell Young, drawing on the work of J. C. Carothers, argued that 'There are well-founded reasons for believing that the incidence of insan-ity in Africans living in their natural environment is low. Higher rates of insanity are found in Africans living away from their former tribal areas, and this section of the community is likely to increase in the future'.[47] More logical reasons for rising admissions, however, were increases in the availability of accommodation, changing socio-economic conditions (particularly in Kampala) which were straining the ability of families to care for the mentally ill, as well as the growth of road networks, which made it easier for the police to transport suspected cases to Kampala. Proximity to the mental hospital was a key factor in admission, with the Ganda, the main ethnic group in and around Kampala, as well as Rwandan immigrants, predominating among inpatients. By living close to an urban centre, these patients were not only more visible to the colo-nial authorities, but could be transported quickly and at minimal cost.[48] As distances became more manageable towards the end of the colonial period, more patients were brought from elsewhere in Uganda. But the Ganda continued to predominate, comprising 153 of the 558 patients within Mulago Mental Hospital at the end of 1956.[49] Indeed, even by the 1960s, a town like Fort Portal, two-hundred miles west of Kampala, had only fifty miles of tarmacked road, creating ongoing reluctance to do anything more than leave suspected mental patients in prison, or cared for at home.[50]

Most patients were brought to the mental hospital following vio-lence, arson or, in urban centres, 'wandering'.[51] This did not mean that the processes of admission were smooth or uncontested, however. Cecil C., a mining engineer who was certified as 'insane' following three weeks of 'alcoholic intemperance' in 1930, was among those who challenged the authority of the police and medical practitioners to diagnose deviant behaviour. While in hospital, according to the official reports, Cecil C. had become aggressive, 'addressing imaginary persons', being 'suspicious of his food', 'filthy' in his habits and 'violent', requiring him 'to be hand-cuffed to his bed'.[52] Addressing the judge presiding over his Reception Order case, Cecil C. argued that these statements were false: 'I was never handcuffed to my bed for filthy habits as I do not possess filthy habits. I am not and never have suffered from hallucinations. I have never been so idiotic as to tear up pieces of paper and distribute them as cheques'.[53] Going further, Cecil C. charged the police who removed him from hospital to Kampala Gaol with ill-treatment:

> On arriving I refused to lie down on the bed. I stood in the doorway with result that I was handcuffed. The cell was locked and I had no attention or a drink for 24 hours. I was never as far as I know reported as being insane. If I was reported, it was done behind my back. In any case there was no second opinion. I therefore resent the reports being made. I shall call the doctors to book. They will have to prove me insane now or face the consequences.[54]

Following the judge's dismissal of Cecil C.'s protestations as to his sanity, he turned his attention to the colonial administration, charging them with undue use of force in restraining him, and threatening legal action. The problem was not so much the ill-treatment, but Cecil C.'s barrage of correspondence, which he kept up much to the consternation of the officials who had to respond to it. Not only did consideration of his claims mean 'time and work for many', but they regarded his 'present attitude' as 'an example of the blackest ingratitude to his custodians', made worse by the fact that he was 'an almost incredible nuisance while under detention...and looking after him was a filthy and horrible business to all concerned'.[55] While, like the judge, the colonial government ultimately refuted the claims of ill-treatment, Cecil C. nevertheless forced them to consider the lack of provision for European patients. Rather than continue to rely on the prison system, there would need to be adequate provision in Mulago Mental Hospital for the short-term confinement of Europeans.

Harold B., a barrister who had been practising in Kampala since his arrival in Uganda in August 1925, evoked similar annoyance among the colonial government with his complaints. Having been arrested on a charge of attempting suicide towards the end of 1928, he had been certified as suffering from 'chronic delusional insanity' and confined in Kampala Gaol before being transferred to Mathari Mental Hospital, Kenya. While it had been usual practice to remove European patients to either Kenya or South Africa, Harold B. made it clear, in increasingly litigious terms, that there was no real legal basis for his transfer or reception in Kenya. While the colonial government admitted, internally, the 'technical illegality of his transfer', they maintained that there was no moral claim to be made: 'He was undoubtedly a madman, and his transfer to the more suitable conditions at Mathari was an act of common humanity'.[56] Shortly after his arrival at Mathari, Harold B. was transferred to South Africa, where he was confined at Fort Napier Institution, Pietermaritzburg. There, his mental state improved sufficiently to justify his discharge, and he soon sought a return to Uganda. The colonial government refused his return request, declaring that his history of insanity made him a 'prohibited immigrant' and potential burden on the state. This did not deter Harold B., however. Drawing on his legal background, Harold B. started to petition the colonial government first for permission to return to Uganda, and second for compensation in the form of a 'compassionate grant'. This correspondence was full of personal appeals, in which he described his record of service during the First World War, as well as how his 'detention as a lunatic has been a horrible mistake and I have lost five years of my life and of my professional career in consequence'.[57] But it was the repeated references to the legal irregularities of his case, as well as the volume of correspondence, which included a petition to the Secretary of State for the Colonies, that created the most annoyance. It was also not wasted effort. While Harold B.'s claims for compensation were unsuccessful, the colonial government not only eventually conceded his return, but provided him with sufficient funds to do so.[58] This did not represent a softening of policy—they fully intended, 'from a practical point of view', to do 'all we can to persuade [him] to go straight to the United Kingdom' and, 'if his circumstances justify it', to start proceedings to remove him from Uganda.[59] Yet Harold B.'s case nevertheless shows that the hard-line stance towards the mentally ill could be successfully challenged.

In contesting decisions relating to their confinement, European patients such as Cecil C. and Harold B. were able to draw on a body of shared knowledge of policy and procedures that would likely have been inaccessible to many of the African patients who made up the majority of psychiatric cases. Even Cecil C., who was aware that he had a right to appeal against his confinement order, complained that he was not allowed to see a legal adviser when he asked to do so.[60] This is not to say that African patients were not able to contest the authority of psychiatry, however; they certainly were, and did so resourcefully. While court and admissions records are lacking, patient records for the CMS Mengo

Hospital, which accepted small numbers of suspected cases of mental illness for examination and short-term treatment, show that African patients were just as unlikely to be passive objects of treatment. Sabakaki, for example, was brought to Mengo Hospital at the end of 1938 by 'people who found him in the road'. While he appeared 'reasonably alert and cooperative', he consistently refused to answer any questions, meaning that no history could be taken. Instead, he lay 'quietly in bed – tho' he has been trying to go away'. Four days later, still refusing to 'give an account of himself', he ran away.[61] While Sabakaki's behaviour could be read as a sign of his irrationality (and it likely was by the doctors at Mengo Hospital), it also represented a refusal to engage in the diagnostic process, and to accept confinement.

The power of psychiatry was further checked by having to negotiate with the families of the mentally ill. This was shown in a case in 1939 when a police officer in western Uganda was unable to detain a suspected lunatic roaming on the property of a European. When the police officer arrived, 'he found his relatives had already taken him away and they had chained him to a piece of wood. For that he could not possibly bring him and they are still guarding him'.[62] The way forward was similarly unclear to those involved in a case in 1954, when a chief described how he wanted to detain a man who was 'a menace to the villagers in his area. He has already attacked a man with a panga and the man is in Kyenjojo Hospital'.[63] His relatives, the chief stressed, 'wish to take him home and guard him'. Uncertain on the correct way to proceed, he asked the police for advice, and sent one of the relatives to explain their case further.[64]

While admission to the mental hospital depended on the judgements of the police and medical practitioners, families played a central role in determining committal, and their reasons for agreeing were often complex. While the Penal Code defined circumstances in which insanity could be used as a defence in criminal trials, relatives could still be pressured into providing compensation for actions taken by the mentally ill. It may have been a fear of such financial and legal responsibility that prompted Paskali B. to implore the District Commissioner (DC) of Toro in 1954 to 'help and send his brother [Alifunsi M.] to Mulago Hospital Kampala where he can be looked after'.[65] He stressed that he was poor, had no wife to assist him and was 'unable to look after the mad man'. As the chief who forwarded his request noted, 'the mad man is doing damage to the property of other people'.[66] He had already killed four cattle, three goats and a dog, burnt a house, and was now 'taking away the property of other people by force'. Not only was there a threat that Alifunsi M. might 'kill people', but 'His brother is poor and asks for help to retain the mad man in jail to stop him damaging the property of other people'.[67] The account hinted at fear of legal action as much as it stressed the burden of care. In requesting assistance, moreover, no distinction was made between confinement in a mental hospital or a jail. Not only did the man associate the activities of his brother with those of criminal lunatics—who despite the existence of Mulago Mental Hospital were still frequently kept in jails for up to a year—but he was keen to be relieved of responsibility for future crimes.[68]

A former chief from Bwamba, near Fort Portal, made similar claims in a letter to the DC Toro in 1960. He noted how his son, Leji W., had recently returned home, having left his wife and destroyed their house and belongings in the process.[69] 'When he returned he was not well', the former chief continued: 'he started to beat people severely....He has beaten all my wives and children and their heads are full of sores caused by his beatings'.[70] In addition, Leji W. had threatened to burn the houses of their neighbours, threatened his father, killed three cattle and caused relatives to flee. The former chief was writing to ask that 'this dangerous mad person may be kept by the Government....One day he will kill a man and the Government will blame me'.[71] The former chief wanted Leji W. to be removed away from home, 'where all people have ran away for fear of him'.[72] Like the previous case, however, he drew no distinction between prison and the asylum—Mulago Mental Hospital was not necessarily a place for treatment, but it was certainly one of confinement, where families might be offered some form of relief from harm, and potential compensation claims.

Even in cases where relatives were aware of the existence of the mental hospital, it is clear from correspondence that they frequently lacked knowledge about the processes of committal. The 'correct' procedure caused some confusion for one man, who attempted to get his father, a former Saza (county) Head Clerk of Kinkizi, committed in 1960. Having written to the District Magistrate, Kigezi, describing how his father 'has now become so dangerous to the community that he has chased my mother, his wife, out of the home', he then contacted the DC Kigezi, to 'obtain necessary forms and detention order [sic.]'.[73] As a teacher, he felt unable to travel to Kabale to make arrangements in person and hoped the forms could be sent to him for completion and then forwarded with the patient. The testimony he provided was deemed to be 'quite useless' by the DC. Detention forms, as the DC noted, were not issued 'at request', but instead followed from a referral by the Saza Chief Kinkizi, the Police Station, Kabale, and the reports of two medical practitioners.[74] Indeed, cases of suspected lunatics were frustrating for district administrators, who were unable to act until the proper procedure had been followed.[75]

In requesting the removal of relatives, families, like the patients themselves, were active agents in mental health care in ways that demanded recognition by the colonial administration. Even if formal requests for certification were unsuccessful, MOs and other officials were aware that they relied upon families to provide extra-institutional care. Patients who exhibited signs of mental illness at the CMS Mengo Hospital, Kampala, for example, might be transferred to Mulago Mental Hospital if they became violent, but this was determined primarily by the willingness and ability of relatives to care for them. Feriteita K., diagnosed with acute syphilitic dementia in 1940, and at Mengo Hospital for just over a month, alternated from being 'stuperous', 'uncomprehending', incontinent, and struggling violently, to 'Cannot be roused to cooperate at all, but not comatose in that she resists attention a little, usually turns over to her left side, sometimes has her eyes open'.[76] In the end, her doctor decided that she was 'too demented to remain in [the] ward': she was defecating on the floor and chewing the bedclothes. Having raised the possibility of a transfer to Mulago Mental Hospital, however, her family decided to take her home.[77] The availability of relatives was just as crucial in a case in 1938, this time involving a twenty-six-year-old female patient, Erivaniy N. Admitted complaining of headache and abdominal pain, she was said to be incapable of answering questions well and exhibited signs of 'mental disturbance', prompting a diagnosis of dementia. Within a day of admission, she suddenly became difficult to manage, with occasional outbursts of being 'Very noisy + uncontrollable'.[78] After three weeks, Erivaniy N. was deemed too 'Noisy + troublesome at night' to remain, and as she had 'apparently no friends' and 'lives alone at home', she was transferred to Mulago.[79] Similarly in 1941, Zalika N., diagnosed with 'acute toxic mania' following malaria, became progressively more unmanageable during her stay in hospital. After a week, she was recorded as being 'Restless, noisy, getting out of bed', and the following day was transferred to Mulago Mental Hospital. Having treated the malaria with quinine, and with no family available, her mental state was too problematic for the mission doctors to discharge her unaccompanied.[80]

It is not difficult to see why patients and their families were reluctant to accept committal to the mental hospital. Across the Uganda Protectorate, people not only had rich languages for mental illness, but a variety of strategies to deal with it—more than it is possible to cover fully here. Herbalists were often 'the first line of defence', living only short distances from patient's homes. When three women 'went mad' near Rukungiri in the late 1950s, according to a local elder, people in his village looked 'for medicinal herbs especially *omwesamuryo* [lit. the one that makes you sneeze] and *olubuya*' and then proceeded to tie them 'to their nose/nostrils'. This, he added, 'would calm them down'.[81] In cases of madness near Lake Kyoga, families 'carved out a tree trunk and inserted in the leg' of the mad person. This tree was called *enkomyo*, meaning literally 'to stop / halt'.[82] Families could also seek the help of a healer who would try to appease the demands of the spirits who had brought on the madness. *Abasawo abaganda* (doctors) in Buganda called the *balubaale* (hero gods), before welcoming and celebrating them within the community.[83] Within these frameworks of healing, patients and families were incorporated into therapies in ways that were neglected by the mental hospital. In the words of one traditional healer, working in Mpigi District, central Uganda, 'with all mental illness, the cause is spiritual and you have to appease and fulfil the ancestors' demands'. Key to success was the role of families and communities, not just in taking part in the treatment, but in acting quickly to prevent the condition from worsening. 'So when one gets a severe madness', she explained, 'the blame is on the parents for failure to fulfil ancestral demands early'.[84] The mental hospital was, in such cases, a last resort, a place for patients who were beyond hope.

PSYCHIATRIC PRACTICES

For many, admission meant long periods of silence and alienation from family networks of care. Not only was the distance and cost of transportation to Kampala prohibitive for most relatives, but communication was less than ideal. An important counterpoint to letters seeking the removal of a violent or difficult family member were requests sent in the months and years following admission, where families enquired about their relatives, often too far away to visit. In 1952, the brother of Kihika B., who had been admitted to Mulago Mental Hospital in 1944, approached the DC Toro to make enquiries into his whereabouts.[85] Having forwarded the enquiry to the Superintendent of Mulago Mental Hospital, the DC Toro was subsequently informed that the patient had died of neurosyphilis six years previously, and was buried at Kololo, Kampala.[86] There was no policy of repatriating bodies, and from the 1930s, those who died at Mulago Mental Hospital were also subject to post-mortem examinations, something at odds with cultural burial practices.[87] In 1954, a similar request was made by two parents for information about their son, Kamugalwire B., who they knew had been admitted to Mulago Mental Hospital the previous year, but about whom they had not received any news. Young replied promptly, but in language that may have been difficult for Kamugalwire B.'s parents to understand. As Young noted, 'His physical health is satisfactory but mentally he is sullen, suspicious retarded [sic.] and without much insight'.[88] Lack of detailed information was also apparent in the response to the request for information made by another father, who reported how his son, Festo M., had run mad the previous year and been taken to Ndorwa Jail, southwest Uganda. While in jail 'his illness increased and he was sent to Mulago Hospital (where mad people are kept). And from then he has never heard of his son'.[89] Festo M. was still alive, Young replied, but stated, briefly, that his behaviour 'is unreliable and his detention is still necessary'.[90]

The communication problems stemmed primarily from a lack of personnel and resources—specialist alienists had no time to compile regular reports on patients' progress—but it was also linked to the unreliability of the information available to administrators, MOs, and the superintendent of the mental hospital. In a case that may not have been uncommon, a police officer in Soroti described his frustration at encountering a suspected lunatic at his local station, who looked lost, perhaps being 'a Muganda or Musoga by tribe'. 'When I try to ask her name', he noted, 'she does not tell me, she said she was not given a name since she was born'.[91] The problems caused by this lack of information could be devastating for both patients and families. Indeed, in July 1930, the DC Toro wrote to the Superintendent, Hoima Lunatic Asylum, to enquire about Zozimu R., who had not been heard of by relatives since being sent to the asylum from Kampala in May.[92] No patient with that name could be found in the asylum registers, however. '[I]f admitted', the Assistant Superintendent noted briefly, 'he may have been described under another name'.[93] No further information about Zozimu R. could be traced in the correspondence—as far as the administration was concerned, he was lost.

For all its claims to benevolence and care, psychiatry lacked the administrative capacity, medical expertise and cultural knowledge to be effective. This was particularly the case before 1949, when Mulago Mental Hospital was under the nominal supervision of J. P. Mitchell, Medical Superintendent of Mulago Hospital, and H. C. Trowell, Specialist Physician, who both had other, more pressing duties at Mulago Hospital and its medical school.[94] But it was hardly much better when Mulago Mental Hospital had on its staff a full-time psychiatrist—first Young from 1949, then Gerald I. Tewfik from 1956. While Young had some experience of psychiatry within a colonial setting, having been Assistant Medical Superintendent of the Lunatic Asylum, Barbados, neither Young nor Tewfik spoke any of the languages in Uganda, relying on vague translations for case histories. They also knew little of the complexities of ideas about mental illness among different ethnic groups or how to understand the behaviours they saw. In this context, it is little surprise that most patients received no formal diagnosis at all. Of 304 patients admitted in the latter half of 1956, Tewfik was able to diagnose only 57, of whom most had an identifiable organic cause (28 were diagnosed with GPI, while 10 were diagnosed with epilepsy).[95] Lacking diagnoses, patients were treated largely symptomatically, with the psychiatrists lacking any clinical control. As Tewfik complained, 'Where electrical treatment was expected to be effective it frequently was not so; many recovered when they were not expected to do so, and others died for no reason known to the psychiatrist or to the pathologist at post mortem'.[96]

From the late 1940s, despite lacking diagnoses, almost all patients would have undergone one of the psychiatric therapies on offer. This included insulin therapy, which may have resulted in deaths due to the inexperience of staff.[97] ECT was also widely employed, with the number under treatment rising from 78 in 1948 to 230 in 1949 to 527 in 1950.[98] And from 1953, Young introduced Largactil and prefrontal leucotomy, something that Young claimed proved useful in 'the most depraved and hopeless cases'.[99] We should not assume that Young did not believe these therapies could offer real hope to patients—they represented the mainstream of psychiatry in the 1950s and 1960s. But they nevertheless served a practical purpose, playing an important role in managing patients who were otherwise difficult to control in a context where there was increasing pressure on accommodation and staff. Leucotomy, in particular, may have had a sedative effect that would have allowed for more patients to be discharged to their families as 'cured'.[100]

Writing about the benefits of the therapies on offer at Mulago Mental Hospital in 1957, Tewfik noted that two patients who had undergone leucotomies were 'greatly improved'.[101] One was a male 'who had been a most difficult patient', but who 'improved markedly and was discharged to the care of his people within two months of operation'. 'The other', Tewfik added, 'is also considerably improved and will be discharged in the near future'.[102]

By 1958, Tewfik also employed chlorpromazine on a regular basis 'in the face of continued strain on accommodation', along with a number of other tranquilizing and sedative drugs 'supplied free by the manufacturers' for the purposes of controlled trials.[103] Yet it was ECT that remained 'by far the most economical method', resulting, 'in suitable cases', in the 'most dramatic and far-reaching results'.[104] In 1957, it was given to 588 patients (the total inpatient population for the year was 662).[105] Most would receive between 4 and 12 treatments each, but a minority of patients received far more.[106] Despite its widespread use, however, Tewfik conceded that it had little effect on the discharge rate, being more 'valuable as a sedative agent'.[107] While no further details are given on these patients, evidence from elsewhere in colonial Africa indicates that these were likely patients who refused to follow the hospital routine, or who exhibited other behaviour that hospital attendants and the psychiatrist interpreted as particularly 'irrational' or difficult. Such was the case with Muchiri R., who was sent from a prison to Mathari Mental Hospital in 1956 'to see if mad'. On arrival, he was reported as being 'Rather turbulent' and 'will not sit down', only agreeing to answer questions 'after being told he will get E.C.T'. While he was not found to be suffering from any obvious mental illness, the admitting doctor, likely psychiatrist Edward Margetts, noted that he would 'ask prison if he is giving any trouble if so E.C.T'. In the following months, Muchiri R. returned to Mathari as an outpatient to receive four rounds of ECT.[108]

With the lack of specialist personnel at Mulago Mental Hospital, much of the day-to-day practice was left to hospital orderlies and attendants. They made observations, administered many of the treatments, and were charged with maintaining order. In 1946, 111 attendants (working in three shift patterns) were assigned to the mental hospital and many would have been required to attend a series of twenty-one lectures given by Baty, with the aid of a Luganda translator, so that 'the mental patients may gain the benefit of skilled treatment'.[109] Topics included a brief celebratory history of psychiatry, as seen at the beginning of this chapter, as well as notes on staff duties, first aid, the classification of mental illness and their symptoms, and observations. 'It is the duty of staff', Baty stressed, 'to observe the patients inside the wards and compounds, and prevent escapes and prevent the patients harming themselves and other patients and to see that the patients are properly cared for and clothed when in the compound'.[110] Above all, staff were to maintain order and discipline, and to act as examples to patients, reflecting the 'moral management' practices that had developed in the UK during the nineteenth century. So, while 'some patients are unusually dirty, attendants should be unusually clean'.[111] They were instructed to be methodical, quiet and calm, and to cheerfully encourage patients to engage in basic 'occupational therapy', including gardening, ward, kitchen and laundry work, needlework, knitting, rug making, cotton growing and pottery.[112]

Throughout the colonial period, such occupational and physical therapies comprised the primary psychiatric treatments on offer at Mulago Mental Hospital. While Young, and his successor from 1956, Gerald I. Tewfik, acknowledged what they saw as an important psychotherapeutic role of traditional healers in treating mental illness, there was no attempt to bring traditional healers into the mental hospital. Yet patients may have drawn on the knowledge and skills of the hospital attendants and orderlies to access traditional forms of healing. At least one hospital attendant at Mulago in the early 1950s had the reputation of having the power of *mayembe* (charms), and worked locally in the parish as a well-known traditional healer and money lender.[113] Notorious for charging 150–200% interest on loans, he was eventually brought before the parish *lukiiko* (council), however, and accused of an act of witchcraft.[114] Certainly, those suffering from mental illness lived within frameworks for understanding mental illness that were completely different from the psychiatrists in charge, and the reliance on hospital attendants and orderlies in the running of the mental hospital may have allowed for flexibility and creativity in treatment.

Routines at Mulago Mental Hospital were strict, with staff reprimanded for breaches. Yet patients still shaped practices within the mental hospital, and lived lives that were not limited to acts of 'resistance'. Patients were constantly 'quarrelling' amongst themselves, making their independence and need for space known to the hospital authorities, who were forced to respond by making provisions for the extension of outside spaces.[115] Those who refused to be confined, moreover, were 'continually escaping by climbing over the fence', not only prompting reassessment of the suitability of railings and hospital accommodation, but taking up time and resources.[116] When the mental hospital was moved to a new site at Butabika, seven miles from Kampala, there was at first no boundary fence at all, and those dissatisfied with the hospital food started to visit the nearby village to request meals.[117] Indeed, food proved a powerful way through which patients made their importance and needs felt. While the hospital authorities dedicated considerable time and effort to ensuring that the mental hospital diet struck a balance between cost, availability and the ideals of colonial nutritional science, the patients made it clear that food had important cultural and social significance that required consideration. As elsewhere in East Africa, food was an important marker of identity, with preparation, presentation and the act of eating representing a form of ritual.[118] Such was the importance of plantains to the Ganda, the largest ethnic group at Mulago Mental Hospital, that the Luganda word for plantains, *matooke*, meant 'food', and represented a point of distinction between the Ganda and other ethnic groups, such as the Nyoro, whose staple food was millet.[119] When, following a period of price inflation and *matooke* shortages in central Uganda in the 1940s and early 1950s, patients were served maize-meal for part of a year, they refused to eat for weeks, contributing to as many as 120 deaths and panic among the hospital authorities.[120] Food mattered, and not for the reasons that the hospital administrators—obsessed with statistics and nutrition—believed that it did.

CONCLUSION

By the time an Australian expatriate psychiatrist, T. W. Murray, was appointed in 1960, the direction of psychiatry was starting to show signs of change. An ambitious scheme to develop psychiatry as a specialism for African doctors was being discussed by Makerere University College and the colonial government. Stephen B. Bosa, Uganda's first psychiatrist, was at the Maudsley Hospital, London, working towards his Diploma in Psychological Medicine (DPM), and the first formal attempt to extend the reach of psychiatry beyond the mental hospital had been made with the opening of a psychiatric ward at Soroti Hospital. Overcrowding at Mulago Mental Hospital, along with pressures on space caused by the expansion of other specialist departments at Mulago Hospital, had also seen plans to move the mental hospital further from Kampala, with access to 1000 acres of land 'to ensure that the inmates have privacy, and can be usefully employed in work that will help in their cure'.[121] The new hospital was built at Butabika, seven miles outside of Kampala, with views over Lake Victoria. It was still in the process of construction when opened to patients in 1955, but by 1964, the final (criminal) patients had been transferred to a new specialist unit, and Mulago Mental Hospital was closed for good. Regarded as something of a parting gift from the British at Independence, Butabika Hospital would be the face of psychiatry during the years of decolonisation.

The growth and organisation of psychiatry in colonial Uganda had been premised on and shaped by more than a singular intention to define and subdue deviant populations. The need for a mental hospital had at first been a practical and moral issue, driven by scandal and the central-ising tendencies of the 1920s, then later framed as a medical concern, with desires to break the association between lunacy and crime and to treat mental illness by 'modern' means. Despite the steady expansion of psychiatry throughout the colonial period, psychiatric practice remained limited: constrained by location, finances and few specialist personnel, psychiatry lacked the geographical reach and therapeutic power to be effective. It was still, for most, a last resort, reserved primarily for the most 'urgent' or difficult cases. In the absence of confidence or certainty in the mental hospital, patients and their families continued to respond to the idea of 'confinement' in different ways. For some, the mental hos-pital was simply a place for the most difficult 'lunatics', little different from a prison, and to be used when the financial responsibility became too great, or the patient too violent. For others, admission to a men-tal hospital was an alienating experience for both patient and family—a place where communication was limited and culturally sanctioned forms of healing could not be formally accessed. Young complained to readers of the *Uganda Argus* in 1955 that there were 'several factors working against the recovery of the mentally sick in Uganda', of which 'the laud-able one of wanting to look after the mentally sick in the family circle as long as possible' was key.[122] He pointed to a 'widely held' belief that had emerged around psychiatry that saw the mental hospital as a place of permanent confinement. This belief, 'built on superstition', held 'that to allow a relative to enter a mental hospital was as good as signing his death warrant'.[123] These perceptions of psychiatry would persist beyond Independence in 1962, proving difficult, if not impossible, for psychia-trists to overcome.

The marginal nature of institutional psychiatry in colonial Uganda has important implications for our understanding of the relationship between psychiatry and decolonisation. Despite ongoing concern about rising numbers of inpatients at Mulago and then Butabika Hospital, in the context of Uganda's total population, which in 1959 stood at an estimated 6.5 million, these numbers were extremely small.[124] Psychiatry was not, then, in a position where it had to face questions of what to do with vast numbers of inpatients, as it would have to do in Europe and the USA in the context of deinstitutionalisation. For all its flaws, moreover, the mental hospital, as the sole face of psychiatry, remained the only institution available to psychiatrists in the years immediately leading up to, and following Independence. Rather than engage in a process of dismantling an institution that had limited geographical and cultural reach, the more pressing question, was how to build up and extend the reach of psychiatry: how to make it culturally relevant, how to help people who lived far from the hospital walls, and how to convince them to turn to psychiatry in times of distress.

NOTES

1. As cited in D. Zeller, 'The Establishment of Western Medicine in Buganda' (Unpublished PhD thesis, Columbia University, 1971), p. 333.
2. Bodleian Library, University of Oxford (BOD) Mss.Afr.s.1872(84) (Papers of Philip William Hutton), ff. 30–31, 'Some Comments on African Attitudes to European Medicine'.
3. BOD Mss.Afr.s.1589 (Papers of Charles Baty), 'Lectures & Treatments', f. 9, 'Lecture 1—On Study', n. d.
4. Ibid.
5. Ibid.
6. M. Vaughan, *Curing Their Ills: Colonial Power and African Illness* (Cambridge, 1991), p. 120.
7. Y. Pringle, 'Crossing the Divide: Medical Missionaries and Government Service in Uganda, 1897–1940', in Anna Greenwood, ed., *Beyond the State: The Colonial Medical Services in British Africa* (Manchester, 2015). See also: J. Kuhanen, *Poverty, Health and Reproduction in Early Colonial Uganda* (Joensuu, 2005).
8. On medical missionaries and mental illness, see Y. Pringle, 'Neurasthenia at Mengo Hospital, Uganda: A Case Study in Psychiatry and a Diagnosis, 1906–50', *The Journal of Imperial and Commonwealth History* 44(2) (2016), pp. 241–262.

9. On medical training in Uganda, see especially J. Iliffe, *East African Doctors: A History of the Modern Profession* (Kampala, 2002); A. M. Odonga, *The First Fifty Years of Makerere Medical School and the Foundation of Scientific Medical Education in East Africa* (Kampala: Marianum Press, 1989).

10. See, for example, the remarks in BOD Mss.Afr.S.1872(144A) (Hugh Trowell Papers), 'Dr. Hugh Trowell OBE, MD, FRCP', p. 12. See also: M. Lyons, 'The Power to Heal: African Medical Auxiliaries in Colonial Belgian Congo and Uganda', in D. Engels and S. Marks, eds., *Contesting Colonial Hegemony: State and Society in Africa and India* (London, 1994).

11. G. C. Beuschel, 'Shutting Africans Away: Lunacy, Race and Social Order in Colonial Kenya, 1910–1963' (Unpublished PhD thesis, SOAS, University of London, 2001), p. 127.

12. A. R. Cook, *Uganda Memories, 1897–1940* (Kampala, 1945), p. 1; W. D. Foster, *The Early History of Scientific Medicine in Uganda* (Nairobi, 1970), pp. 93–107; D. M. Haynes, 'Framing Tropical Disease in London: Patrick Manson, *Filaria Perstans*, and the Uganda Sleeping Sickness Epidemic, 1891–1902', *Social History of Medicine* 13(3) (2000), pp. 467–493; D. Neill, 'Paul Ehrlich's Colonial Connections: Scientific Networks and Sleeping Sickness Drug Therapy Research, 1900–1914', *Social History of Medicine* 22(1) (2008), pp. 61–77.

13. K. A. Hoppe, *Lords of the Fly: Sleeping Sickness Control in British East Africa, 1900–1960* (Westport, CN, 2003), p. 1. On the development of the Colonial Medical Service in Uganda during this period, see A. Beck, *A History of the British Medical Administration of East Africa: 1900–1950* (Cambridge, MA, 1970), Ch. 2.

14. The National Archives, Kew, United Kingdom (TNA) CO 536/32, 62 (Blue Book + Report, 1908–1909).

15. A. R. Cook, 'A Visit to a Branch Dispensary and a Sleeping Sickness Camp in Uganda', *Mercy and Truth* 148 (1909), p. 108.

16. BOD Mss.Afr.s.1091 Box 3 File 1 (Baker Papers), f. 11, 'A Night and Day in a "Sleeping Sickness" Camp', p. 3.

17. TNA CO 536/31, 38571 (Sleeping Sickness), 'Official Report on the Measures Adopted by the Uganda Administration in Dealing with "Sleeping Sickness" in the Protectorate, 17 November 1909', para. 52.

18. TNA CO 536/6 no. 49 (Report on the Bankruptcy and Lunacy Ordinance, 1906). In this year, four people were certified as insane under the new legislation. TNA CO 536/14 no. 110 (Report on Legal Dept. 1906. Judge Carter), p. 3.

19. TNA CO 536/6 no. 49 (Ordinance No. 4 1906 "Bankruptcy and Lunacy" Submits). Also TNA CO 536/2 no. 61 ([1] Sergt J. Sayers,

Inspr of Police. [2] Sergt Pugh, Inspr of Police), Medical Certificate
dated 5 June 1905.
20. TNA CO 536/8 no. 207, letter from H. Hesketh Bell, H.M.
Commissioner, to the Earl of Elgin and Kincardine, 1 November 1906,
p. 1.
21. TNA CO 536/8 no. 207, letter from H. Hesketh Bell, H.M.
Commissioner, to the Earl of Elgin and Kincardine, 1 November 1906,
pp. 1–3.
22. TNA CO 536/163/2; TNA CO 536/165/18; TNA CO 822/76/12
(Lunacy).
23. Uganda National Archives (UNA) A46/1120 (Hoima Prison: Leper
and Lunatic Prisoners), letter from Captain Chiddick, Commissioner of
Prisons, Kampala, to Chief Secretary, Entebbe, 24 July 1913.
24. TNA CO 536/62 no. 42541 (Prisons—Inspection Report 1912),
'Report of the Inspector General of Police and Prisons on the Uganda
Government Prisons for the Year 1912', para. 2.
25. Uganda Protectorate, *Blue Book for the Year Ended 31st March, 1915*
(Entebbe, 1915), p. Da1; TNA CO 536/104 no. 604 (Death Rate
among Prisoners), letter from C. A. Wiggins to Chief Secretary,
Entebbe, 30 September 1920; TNA CO 536/104 no. 604, 'Report on
Lunatic Asylum, Hoima', p. 3.
26. Uganda Protectorate, *Annual Medical and Sanitary Report for the Year
Ended 31st December, 1923* (Entebbe, 1924), pp. 9–10.
27. Beck, *A History of the British Medical Administration*, Ch. 4; C. P.
Youe, 'Peasants, Planters and Cotton Capitalists: The "Dual Economy"
of Uganda', *Canadian Journal of African Studies* 12(2) (1978), pp.
163–184.
28. Pringle, 'Crossing the Divide.'
29. On attempts to combat venereal disease, see especially C. Summers,
'Intimate Colonialism: The Imperial Production of Reproduction in
Uganda, 1907–1925', *Signs* 16(4) (1991), pp. 787–807; M. W. Tuck,
'Syphilis, Sexuality, and Social Control: A History of Venereal Disease in
Colonial Uganda' (Unpublished PhD thesis, Northwestern University,
1997). On the staffing of the Colonial Medical Service more generally, see A. Crozier, *Practising Colonial Medicine: The Colonial Medical
Service in British East Africa* (London, 2007).
30. UNA C1266 (Medical Organisation of Medical Units at Kampala),
memorandum by Major Keane entitled 'Asiatic Hospital—Kampala',
May 1928. Such was the importance of the tendency towards centralisation that in 1936 officials considered relocating the Medical
Headquarters from Entebbe to Kampala. See UNA J1/23 (Medical
Headquarters—Transfer of, to Kampala).

31. UNA C0524 (Miscellaneous—Lunatics, Death of, in Kampala Jail); A. R. Dunbar, *A History of Bunyoro-Kitara* (Nairobi, 1965), pp. 121–122.
32. Albert Cook Memorial Library, Makerere University (ACMM), Mengo Hospital Correspondence, letter from Major Keane, Director of Medical and Sanitary Services, Entebbe, Uganda, to Dr. Cook, 11 September 1930.
33. Ibid.
34. Ibid.
35. Uganda Protectorate, *Annual Report of the Medical Department for the Year Ended 31st December, 1930* (Entebbe, 1931), p. 47.
36. J. Sadowsky, *Imperial Bedlam: Institutions of Madness in Colonial Southwest Nigeria* (Berkeley and Los Angeles, 1999), Ch. 2.
37. 'A Lunatic at Large', *Uganda Herald*, 3 July 1935, p. 10.
38. Kabale District Archives (KDA) (Circulars), circular memorandum from Chief Secretary entitled 'Mulago Mental Hospital, 25 March 1936'; Mountains of the Moon University, Fort Portal (MMU) MED 1079(295) (Lunatics), f. 1, circular memorandum from J. Hope Reford to all Medical Officers, 8 December 1926; Soroti District Archives (SDA) JUD 1/2 (Lunatics), f. 22, letter from J. S. Champion, Ministry of Health and Medical Headquarters, Entebbe, to M. Rogers, DC Teso, 31 March 1960; ACMM, Medical Department Circulars, circular memorandum entitled 'Admissions to Mental Hospitals', 20 November 1957.
39. MMU MED 1079(295), f. 1, circular memorandum from J. Hope Reford to all Medical Officers, 8 December 1926.
40. UNA D107/12 (Lunatics: Transport of Mental Patients), ff. 4–5, letter from Lieut.-Colonel, Commissioner of Police, to Director of Medical Services, Entebbe, 10 February 1942.
41. 'Eddwaliro Ly'abalalu', *Gambuze*, 6 January 1933, p. 2.
42. 'Notes by the Way: A Weekly Commentary on Current Affairs', *Uganda Herald*, Wednesday 14 August 1935, p. 13.
43. J. F. Wood, 'A Half Century of Growth in Ugandan Psychiatry', *Uganda Atlas of Disease Distribution* (Kampala, 1968), p. 118.
44. Uganda Protectorate, *Annual Report of the Medical Department for the Year Ended 31st December, 1956* (Entebbe, 1957), p. 49.
45. Uganda Protectorate, *Annual Report of the Medical Department for the Year ended 31st December, 1938* (Entebbe, 1939), p. 55; Uganda Protectorate, *Annual Report of the Medical Department, 1956*, p. 49.
46. See, for example, G. I. Tewfik, 'Mulago Hospital Clinical Staff Meeting April 26, 1958: The African Mind Fact or Myth?' *East African Medical Journal* 35(8) (1958), pp. 512–513.

47. Uganda Protectorate, *Annual Report of the Medical Department for the Year Ended 31st December, 1951* (Entebbe, 1952), p. 60.
48. UNA D107/12, ff. 4–5, letter from Lieut.-Colonel, Commissioner of Police, to Director of Medical Services, Entebbe, 10 February 1942.
49. Uganda Protectorate, *Annual Report of the Medical Department, 1956*, p. 49.
50. H. G. Egdell, 'A Rural Psychiatric Service in Uganda', *Psychopathologie Africaine* 6(1) (1970), p. 89.
51. G. I. Tewfik, 'Problems of Mental Illness in Uganda', *Mental Disorders and Mental Health in Africa South of the Sahara: CCTA/CSA-WFMH-WHO Meeting of Specialists on Mental Health* (Bukavu, 1958), p. 63.
52. TNA CO 536/165/18, f. 91, 'Medical Certificate'.
53. TNA CO 536/165/18, f. 86, 'Enclosure K' of Lunacy Cause No. 12 of 1930, p. 2.
54. TNA CO 536/165/18, f. 87, 'Enclosure K' of Lunacy Cause No. 12 of 1930, p. 3.
55. TNA CO 536/165/18, ff. 95–98, letter to the Chief Secretary's Office, Entebbe, 23 April 1931.
56. TNA CO 536/179/1, f. 7, note by J. S. Macpherson, 1 November 1933.
57. TNA CO 536/179/1, ff. 43–45, letter dated 6 September 1933.
58. TNA CO 536/179/1, ff. 39–42, letter from the Governor of Uganda, 3 October 1933.
59. TNA CO 536/179/1, f. 4, note by Mr. Duncan.
60. TNA CO 536/165/18, ff. 56–60, 'Enclosure A'.
61. ACMM, Mengo Hospital Case Notes, 1938, Vol. 8, No. 2157, p. 647.
62. MMU 471(118) (Loc Govt—Lunatics & Vagrants), f. 48, letter addressed to DC Toro, 14 April 1939; MMU 471(118), f. 47, letter from DC Toro, 11 April 1939.
63. MMU JUD 4(1) (Lunacy), f. 22, letter addressed to O.C. Police, Toro, 13 September 1954.
64. Ibid.
65. MMU JUD 4(1), f. 26, letter addressed to DC Toro, 21 September 1954.
66. Ibid.
67. Ibid.
68. Uganda Protectorate, *Annual Report on the Treatment of Offenders for the Year Ended 31st December, 1954* (Entebbe, 1955), pp. 13–14.
69. MMU JUD 4(1), f. 127, letter addressed to DC Toro, 15 June 1960.
70. Ibid.
71. Ibid.
72. Ibid.

73. Kabale District Archives (KDA) JUD 1/3 I (Lunacy), f. 247, letter addressed to DC Kigezi, 29 October 1960.
74. KDA JUD 1/3 I, f. 248, letter from DC Kigezi, 3 November 1960.
75. MMU 471(118), f. 46, letter from DC Toro to Katikiro of Toro, 26 July 1938.
76. ACMM, Mengo Hospital Case Notes, 1940, Vol. 4, No. 1175, p. 707.
77. Ibid.
78. ACMM, Mengo Hospital Case Notes, 1938, Vol. 4, No. 1009, p. 347.
79. Ibid.
80. ACMM, Mengo Hospital Case Notes, 1941, Vol. 5, No. 1629.
81. Interview with Ankole male, approximately 71 years old (RUK-06), Butinde Village, Kebisoni Sub-County, Rukungiri District, 5 July 2011.
82. Interview with Ganda male, approximately 92 years old (KAY-03), Kawuku, Kayunga District, 3 June 2011.
83. J. Orley, *Culture and Mental Illness* (Nairobi, 1970), pp. 20–24; N. Kodesh, 'Networks of Knowledge: Clanship and Collective Well-Being in Buganda', *The Journal of African History* 49(2) (2008), pp. 197–216.
84. Interview conducted with P. Nabuto (MPG-04), Buyijja, Mpigi District, 19 October 2011.
85. MMU JUD 4(1), f. 11, letter from DC Toro to Superintendent, Mental Hospital, Mulago, 4 December 1952.
86. MMU, JUD 4(1), f. 12, copy of letter from Medical Superintendent, Mulago, to DC Toro, 2 August 1946.
87. Post-mortem examinations were conducted for research purposes. See, for example, W. R. Billington, 'Neurosyphilis in Natives of East Africa' (Unpublished MD thesis, University of Cambridge, 1945).
88. KDA JUD 1/3 I, f. 29, letter from G. Campbell Young to DC Kigezi, 4 January 1954.
89. KDA JUD 1/3 I, f. 4, letter from Yeremiya Bigombe, for Saza Chief Ndorwa, to DC Kigezi, 10 May 1954.
90. KDA JUD 1/3 I, f. 7, letter from G. Campbell Young to DC Kigezi, 19 May 1954.
91. SDA JUD 1/2, f. 26, letter addressed to O.C. Police, Soroti Teso, 8 April 1960.
92. MMU MED 1079(295), f. 98, letter from DC Toro to Superintendent, Lunatic Asylum, Hoima, 11 July 1930; MMU MED 1079(295), f. 97, note addressed to DC Toro, 8 July 1930.

93. MMU MED 1079(295), f. 99, letter from Assistant Superintendent, Mental Hospital, to DC Toro, 18 July 1930.

94. BOD Mss.Afr.s.1872(144B) (Hugh Trowell Papers), 'Transcript of Conversations Between Hugh Trowell and Elizabeth Bray', p. 34; BOD Mss.Afr.s.1589, 'Correspondence—Uganda Govt.', letter from Crown Agents, London to Charles Baty, 9 March 1940.

95. G. I. Tewfik, 'Psychoses in Africa', *Mental Disorders and Mental Health in Africa South of the Sahara: CCTA/CSA-WFMH-WHO Meeting of Specialists on Mental Health* (Bukavu, 1958), p. 131.

96. Ibid., p. 127

97. Uganda Protectorate, *Annual Report of the Medical Department, 1956*, p. 49.

98. Uganda Protectorate, *Annual Report of the Medical Department for the Year Ended 31st December, 1950* (Entebbe, 1951), p. 31.

99. Uganda Protectorate, *Annual Report of the Medical Department for the Year Ended 31st December, 1954* (Entebbe, 1955), p. 36.

100. J. D. Pressman, *Last Resort: Psychosurgery and the Limits of Medicine* (San Francisco, 1998).

101. Uganda Protectorate, *Annual Report of the Medical Department for the Year Ended 31st December, 1957* (Entebbe, 1958), p. 46.

102. *Annual Report of the Medical Department for 1957*, p. 46.

103. Uganda Protectorate, *Annual Report of the Medical Department for the Year Ended 31st December, 1958* (Entebbe, 1959), p. 61.

104. Uganda Protectorate, *Annual Report of the Medical Department, 1958*, p. 61.

105. G. I. Tewfik, 'Problems of Mental Illness in Uganda', p. 68.

106. G. I. Tewfik, 'Low Incidence of Fractures Among Africans Following Electro-Convulsive Therapy', *West African Medical Journal* 9(1) (1960), p. 26.

107. Tewfik, 'Psychoses in Africa', p. 134.

108. Mathari Hospital Records Project, Nairobi, AF/M.132/55.

109. BOD Mss.Afr.s.1589, 'Lectures & Treatments', f. 12, 'Lecture 1'.

110. BOD Mss.Afr.s.1589, 'Lectures & Treatments', f. 13, 'Objects of the Mental Hospital'.

111. BOD Mss.Afr.s.1589, 'Lectures & Treatments', f. 11, 'Chief Duties of Attendants'.

112. UNA J142 (Mental Hospital: Occupational Therapy for the Treatment of Patients); Uganda Protectorate, *Annual Report of the Medical Department for the Year Ended 31st December, 1937* (Entebbe, 1938),

p. 51; Uganda Protectorate, *Annual Report of the Medical Department for the Year Ended 31st December, 1946* (Entebbe, 1949), pp. 48–49; Uganda Protectorate, *Annual Report of the Medical Department for the Year Ended 31st December, 1948* (Entebbe, 1950), p. 48; Uganda Protectorate, *Annual Report of the Medical Department, 1949*, p. 44.

113. A. W. Southall and P. C. W. Gutkind, *Townsmen in the Making: Kampala and Its Suburbs* (Kampala, 1957), p. 206.

114. Ibid., pp. 149–150.

115. BOD Mss.Afr.s.1589, 'Correspondence', ff. 26–30, letter from Mental Hospital, Mulago, to Director of Medical Services, Entebbe, 31 October 1946, p. 1.

116. Ibid.

117. Interview with two Ganda females (BUT-01), Butabika, 16 May 2011; Interview with Ganda male (BUT-03), Butabika, 23 May 2011; Interview with Ganda female (BUT-04), Butabika, 23 June 2011.

118. See M. Graboyes, 'Chappati Complaints and Biriani Cravings: The Aesthetics of Food in Colonial Zanzibari Institutions', *Journal of Eastern African Studies* 5(2) (2011), pp. 313–328.

119. J. J. Jørgensen, *Uganda: A Modern History* (London, 1981), p. 37.

120. Uganda Protectorate, *Annual Report of the Medical Department, 1954*, p. 36.

121. BOD Mss.Afr.s.1589, 'Correspondence', ff. 17–18, 'Extract from Report and Recommendation on the Post-War Development of the Medical Services', p. 1.

122. '£90,000 Hospital Wing at Butabika Opened', *Uganda Argus*, 11 June 1955, p. 5.

123. Ibid.

124. Uganda Government, *The First Five-Year Development Plan* (Entebbe, 1962), p. 2.

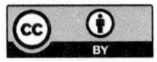

CHAPTER 3

The 'Africanisation' of Psychiatry

As preparations for decolonisation started to accelerate after the Second World War, the need for knowledge on what was 'normal' and 'abnormal' in the African was increasingly noted. 'We need extensive research on African mental health not in the future but now', claimed Donald Mackay, mission doctor in Northern Rhodesia: 'We need mental clinics in every township. We need men trained in psychiatry and steeped in African background to stem the tide of threatening maladjustment. We hear much of development—but where is there development so pressing as this'.[1] Most European doctors, Mackay stressed, were ignorant about psychiatric and psychological medicine: 'The neurosis, the small maladjustment, have passed us by', meaning psychiatry was limited to 'when some obstreperous lunatic is certified and packed away to some Institution, dead to the world of his fellows'.[2] Yet the 'mental consequences' of 'detribalisation', as articulated by those in the East African School of Psychiatry and Psychology, were inescapable: 'time waits for no master. If we do not face the problem now, and deal with maladjusted individuals, the problem will face us in another generation and we shall have a maladjusted nation to deal with'.[3] In Mackay's opinion, the subject was best approached by 'hard grinding study' of the African's 'background, his faiths, his hopes, his fears, his sex life—and everything that makes up the mosaic of his mental environment'.[4] Others, however, contended that Africans were better placed to understand what was 'normal' and 'abnormal'. Responding to Mackay in 1948, John A. Carman, editor

© The Author(s) 2019
Y. Pringle, *Psychiatry and Decolonisation in Uganda*,
Mental Health in Historical Perspective,
https://doi.org/10.1057/978-1-137-60095-0_3

of the *East African Medical Journal*, argued that because of the complex variations in African mentality and 'the hidden secrets of the hills and forests', 'the right type of African doctor is the only person who can hope to approach the subject in the proper way'.[5]

What constituted the 'right type' of African doctor had long been debated in East Africa—not least in Kenya, where Europeans feared that African doctors would 'get too big for their boots'.[6] In Uganda, the colonial government was more open to the technical training of Africans, including through their own medical programme at Makerere Medical School, based at Mulago Hospital, which accepted students from across East Africa. While the interest in medical training set Uganda apart from Kenya, it should be remembered that Africans did not receive equal status as doctors until 1951, being, as John Iliffe has stressed, 'merely assistants, embittered by subordinate status and unrewarding conditions of work'.[7] Colonial officials also frequently justified the extending of training to Africans on the basis of notions of cultural difference. W. H. Kauntze, Director of Medical Services (DMS), noted on the training of sanitation officers in 1937 that 'A European can never quite look at matters from the African point of view....Hence the prime essential is to build up an enlightened body of Africans who can be taught to appreciate the scientific reasons lying behind sanitary law, and who will have such an intimate knowledge of the African mind that the cogent arguments which can be brought forward in favour of sanitary ideals can be so framed as to find favour in spite of inherited beliefs'.[8]

As African doctors started to come together as a professional group in the run-up to Independence in 1962, these ideas did not disappear, but were reworked as political claims to knowledge and status. Opening an article on African patients, Eria M. Babumba noted that he 'was brought up among his own people and knows what his fellow Africans are likely to think, their old beliefs and superstitions, and their usual fears'.[9] The Makerere Medical Graduates' Association, too, argued that African doctors, by right of birth, had 'more direct communication with our fellow African than any other people....Patients trust us more'.[10] Such sentiments were supported by contemporary medical thinking about the importance of psychology in doctor–patient relationships. Addressing the Uganda branch of the British Medical Association (BMA) in 1955, H. C. Trowell described how with his own African patients, 'I seldom feel really at home and I feel sorry for my students that they see this travesty of a physician, one who cannot really talk fluently with his patients and even then has almost no understanding of the medley of motives, hopes, fears, reserves and evasions which are encountered in our African patients'.[11] 'I often wish', he added, 'my students could see me practising among my own people, among whom I detect more quickly the anxieties and background of every case'.[12] In Trowell's opinion, Africans possessed natural cultural 'insight' into their patients' fears and anxieties that could be harnessed through medical training, just as doctors in Europe might come to 'detect' these signs in their own patients.

In the decades following the Second World War, calls for further research into mental illness and the training of Africans in psychiatry coincided with the 'Africanisation' of British colonial rule in Africa. Officially initiated in Uganda in 1952, Africanisation consisted of policies aimed at increasing the number of Africans in the administration through training and promotion. Such policies, which had the most visible effects in the army, the police and the legislative council, were intended to allow Africans to 'stand on their own feet without support, to manage their own affairs without supervision, and to determine their own future for themselves'.[13] Within medicine, Uganda's colonial government attempted to accelerate the process through increased funding for postgraduate training from 1957. In 1960, the first African doctor was appointed to Medical Headquarters, and in 1962, Ivan Kadama became Chief Medical Officer of the newly independent Ministry of Health.[14] Within psychiatry, Stephen B. Bosa, who had worked at Mulago Mental Hospital since 1948, was promoted to consultant psychiatrist in 1961 and finally made head of mental health services in 1964. Africanisation was not revolutionary, however. Nor should it be equated with a decolonisation of psychiatry. Africanisation was a slow devolutionary process that concerned staffing—a transitionary period intended to be good for social, economic and political development, rather than a concession of independence.[15] It also entailed little immediate change in psychiatric practice and organisation. As I show in this chapter, even in his newly promoted position, Bosa was unable to convince those at the Ministry of Health to act on his proposals for psychiatry. When Makerere Medical School decided to open a Department of Psychiatry in 1966, moreover, the new curriculum was modelled along English lines.

This chapter, and the one that follows, is concerned with the experiences of African doctors and psychiatrists as they took over responsibility for psychiatry at the end of empire. Much of this concerns training, from the inclusion of psychiatry on the syllabus at Makerere Medical

School and the use of Mulago Mental Hospital for short-term placements, to the overseas training of Uganda's first psychiatrists, Bosa and
Benjamin H. Kagwa, and to the programmes implemented by Makerere
Medical School in the years following the opening of the Department
of Psychiatry. But it is also concerned with the place of Ugandans, first
within the institutions and structures governing psychiatry during colonial rule, and then in the mental hospital in the early 1960s. Ugandan
doctors were not isolated from local or nationalist politics; indeed, as
became clear during widespread disturbances in the 1940s, they were
often at the centre of it. The Africanisation of psychiatry between the
1940s and the 1960s thus reveals not only an uneasy relationship
between psychiatry and colonial politics, but also the practical difficulties
facing Ugandan psychiatrists at the end of empire.

UGANDA'S FIRST PSYCHIATRISTS

Psychiatry was included in the curriculum at Makerere Medical School
from the outset. Just as medical education in England had by the 1920s
incorporated psychiatry and psychological medicine as compulsory, if
minor, elements of the Bachelor of Medicine degree, so it was considered a necessary part of the medical course in Uganda.[16] In practice,
however, training in psychiatry depended on the ability and availability
of a willing tutor. While in 1946, Philip Hutton, Physician at Mulago
Hospital, gave lectures on neurology, psychiatry and therapeutics, in
the following year, his absence from Mulago Hospital necessitated the
removal of psychiatry from the syllabus altogether.[17] In line with the
practical emphasis of training at Makerere Medical School, which used
Mulago Hospital as a teaching hospital, the mental hospital also acted
as a training ground for psychiatry and psychiatric nursing. From the
early 1940s, a small number of African Medical Officers (AMOs) were
assigned to Mulago Mental Hospital for periods of up to a few months.
In addition to assisting in the routine physical and mental examination of all new patients, they made regular notes on the mental progress of patients and administered specialist treatments.[18] Charles Baty,
Superintendent of Mulago Mental Hospital in the early 1940s, kept
detailed notes on a range of procedures, including electroconvulsive
therapy (ECT), and it is likely these were used for training purposes.
    Medical training created a new group of individuals through which
psychiatry was able to operate in Uganda. While their knowledge of

psychiatry and psychology was limited, it was hardly any less than that of most European medical officers (MOs), whose medical training and lack of cultural knowledge had left them ill-prepared for the types of mental illness they would face in their daily practice.[19] As the number of graduates grew, AMOs also formed an increasingly prominent part of the Colonial Medical Service. While as a group of graduates they remained small until the 1960s, by the late 1930s, their numbers had begun to rival those of European MOs. In 1938, there were 31 AMOs (then called Senior African Medical Assistants) working in government service alongside 33 MOs, 5 Senior MOs, and an assortment of hospital superintendents, surgeons and administrators.[20] Such was the reliance on AMOs, particularly in remote out-stations, that in 1938 the colonial administration granted them limited powers in the certification of mental illness. In a move that was unique in British colonial Africa at the time, the 1938 Mental Treatment Ordinance allowed registered African and Indian medical practitioners to provide one of the two medical reports required by a magistrate, the other being provided by a licensed European practitioner. This amendment, it was noted, was necessary to provide 'more protection to the public', as 'in a number of outstations it would be impossible to assemble two registered practitioners quickly'.[21] In practice, it meant that while Europeans retained a superior status as 'licensed' doctors, responsibility for the mentally ill was increasingly devolved to the new group of Western-trained African doctors. It is unlikely that this had any noticeable effect on diagnosis or treatment, however. With most AMOs originating from Buganda until the 1950s, and lacking language skills in the diverse and often remote areas to which they were posted, problems of communication remained.[22]

While AMOs were exposed to psychiatry and psychological medicine, specialisation in psychiatry was not encouraged. This reflected the lack of regard for psychiatry among Europeans in Uganda, who felt that even short-term placements at Mulago mental hospital 'may not be in the best interests of the A.M.O.' due to its low status, poor working conditions and lack of resources.[23] But it was also indicative of more general restrictions placed on AMOs, who were not offered opportunities for progression or specialisation until after the Second World War. The first Ugandan doctor to qualify in psychiatry did so not in Uganda, or even in the UK, but in the USA. In 1928, Benjamin H. Kagwa, son of Paulo Bakunga, a former Mukwenda (chief of Singo county), left Uganda, travelling first to France and England, before continuing to America in pursuit of higher education.[24] Kagwa later noted that he had been inspired to study medicine by observing Church Missionary Society (CMS) doctors Albert, Jack and Ernest Cook while at Mengo High School, Kampala. 'Their mannerisms, friendliness, apparatus, and handling of patients', he recalled, 'as well as their seeming omniscience, had him spellbound'.[25]

With financial support from his father, the Buganda Kingdom, and the Phelps-Stokes Fund, Kagwa studied at Lincoln, Columbia, and New York Universities, gaining an MD in 1940.[26] As he approached his graduation, however, the colonial government informed him that they would not recognise his American qualifications. If he decided to return to Uganda, he would be registered as an African Assistant Medical Officer (AAMO), the highest position an African medical practitioner could hope to achieve in Uganda at the time, but would not be registered as a doctor. Any higher position, it was noted, would undermine efforts to promote Uganda's own diploma in medicine which, following the recommendations of the 1937 de la Warr Commission, it was hoped would one day be recognised as a full medical degree by the British General Medical Council (GMC).[27] The absurdity of the situation was highlighted by J. E. W. Flood, Director of Colonial Scholars, in December 1939, when he complained that 'it occurs to me that the Uganda Government is simply being sticky for stickiness' sake. It is a perfectly lunatic situation that a black gentleman wearing a string of beads and a smile can practise "native medicine" if he likes, but poor Kagwa, who is a highly educated gentleman, would not be allowed to practise even with the M. D. of New York University unless he cares to set up as a "native" practitioner'.[28]

Refusing to accept these conditions of return, Kagwa went on to complete residencies in neuropsychiatry at the Homer G. Phillips Hospital, St. Louis, as well as Chicago, before finally settling in New York.[29] According to Kagwa, he had been drawn to psychiatry in the second year of his medical degree when he had accompanied the Viennese psychiatrist and neurologist Paul Schilder on ward rounds at New York's Bellevue Hospital. Kagwa recalled a 'tantalizing' case involving an elderly chronic alcoholic white male, from whom he and a fellow student were able to elicit 'random ideas and fantastic yarns'.[30] Yet it was the 'scientific exactness' of clinical neurology, he later decided, that drew him to neuropsychiatry.[31] Over the next twenty-five years, Kagwa worked variously as a psychiatrist, electroencephalographer and neurologist at a range of hospitals in New York, and became an active member of the

Manhattan Central Medical Society, the New York Neurological Society, the American Academy of Neurology, the Brooklyn Psychiatric Society, as well as the American Medical Association, among other bodies.[32] At a time when his colleagues in Uganda were still fighting for recognition of their qualifications and status, Kagwa was establishing a reputation for himself as a neuropsychiatric expert.

Kagwa may have been the first Ugandan to qualify as a psychiatrist, but he was not the first to practise in Uganda. That title goes to Bosa, who received his medical diploma from Makerere in 1945, started work as an AMO attached to Mulago Mental Hospital in 1948 and received a Diploma in Psychological Medicine (DPM) from the Maudsley Hospital in 1961.[33] The decision to appoint an AMO to Mulago Mental Hospital on a full-time basis originated in a report by J. C. Carothers, who had visited in early 1943 on the request of the colonial government. Carothers was tasked with reporting on existing arrangements for mental patients and to suggest ways of ensuring uniformity in psychiatric provision across East Africa, particularly in the legal and practical arrangements for European lunatics.[34] Carothers' report confirmed much of what the medical authorities in Uganda already knew: the mental hospital was overcrowded, the accommodation inadequate (particularly for European cases, who were still held for short periods prior to being transferred to Kenya or South Africa), and specialist therapies lacking.[35] But it also raised the question of the appointment of a full-time (European) Specialist Alienist to take over as Superintendent of Mulago Mental Hospital. While they were being recruited, Carothers added, an AMO would be welcomed at Mathari Mental Hospital, Kenya, for training as a Hospital Assistant.[36] J. P. Mitchell, Medical Superintendent of Mulago Hospital, with responsibility for Mulago Mental Hospital and Makerere Medical School, took issue with these last two points. Rather than appointing a European directly to the hospital, he argued that 'an interested A.M.O. would suffice'. Not only was the treatment available at Mulago Mental Hospital limited, but there were not enough European patients to justify the appointment of a specialist.[37] Mitchell was also keen for the AMO to take on more than the assistant role Carothers had in mind. His views were indicative of more general attitudes towards medical education in Uganda, which in the 1940s saw Makerere Medical School raise entry standards and revise the curriculum with a view to securing recognition for the medical diploma by the British GMC.[38]

In October 1948, Bosa was selected among the AMOs at Mulago Hospital for the new position at Mulago Mental Hospital. By 1948, Bosa was working full time in the women's wards at Mulago Hospital, where he was described as 'competent' but liable to carelessness, for which he was reprimanded on at least one occasion.[39] Considering the reports against him, Bosa's transfer to mental work may be seen as a punishment, as career prospects for AMOs at Mulago Mental Hospital were almost non-existent. He had aptitude and an interest in the work, however, and by 1955 had decided to pursue postgraduate study. Studying abroad was an ambition of many of East Africa's doctors during the 1950s. A small number of scholarships had been available from the late 1940s for postgraduate study in the UK, expanding from the mid-1950s as the Africanisation of the colonial administration got underway and as GMC recognition afforded more opportunities for African doctors in British medical schools. With the exception of experiments in postgraduate surgery, studying abroad remained the only way to secure a postgraduate qualification through the 1950s.[40] Bosa was no exception in his desire to specialise. Clearly aware that his position as the only African doctor willing to work at Mulago Mental Hospital gave him power to negotiate his future, Bosa made postgraduate study a condition of him continuing to work with the mentally ill. If studying abroad was not possible, Bosa stressed to the Medical Department in 1955, 'he wished to be posted away from the Mental Hospital back into some hospital where he could do general medicine'.[41] While AMOs were not usually given a choice about their location, they were able to leave and go into more lucrative private practice from 1949, something that led to an exodus from the Colonial Medical Service during the 1950s.[42]

In December 1955, Bosa travelled on a government scholarship to the Institute of Psychiatry at the Maudsley Hospital, London, to embark on the DPM. By 1955, he already had extensive experience of all forms of treatment used at Mulago Mental Hospital, including ECT, insulin shock therapy, leucotomy, drug abreaction and antipsychotic drugs.[43] Having had no information about the course or life in London, however, he reported feeling bewildered on arrival. The problem stemmed in part from the fact that, due to lack of staff at Mulago Mental Hospital, he had only been granted a period of one year's leave in order to complete a two-year course. As D. L. Davies, Dean of the Institute of Psychiatry, noted in 1957, Bosa was a good student and appeared 'very happy with the instruction he has had', but had been required to attend first- and second-year lectures at the same time.[44] Perhaps unsurprisingly due to the pressure on his time, Bosa failed to pass Part I of the examinations. While Bosa's scholarship was later extended to cover the full two years of the course, he was at a disadvantage because it had never been made clear to him that what was required was 'wide reading with relatively superficial knowledge, rather than [a] sound grasp of fundamental principles'.[45] Bosa returned to London in November 1959 to retake the DPM, which he was awarded in 1961.[46]

The inclusion of Bosa and other AMOs within the formal institutions and structures of psychiatry comprised only a minor part of the Africanisation of the colonial administration in the 1940s and 1950s. Most AMOs continued to have only a rudimentary knowledge of psychiatry, despite facing cases of mental illness in clinics and hospitals across the country. Yet their presence is important for our understanding of the relationship between psychiatry and politics at the end of empire. This came to the fore in the political dissent that erupted in Buganda in the 1940s. The attempted removal from office in 1944 of Samwiri Wamala, *Katikiro* (prime minister) of Buganda, on the grounds that he was suffering from a serious mental disorder, and the involvement of Bosa in public disturbances in 1949, point to an ambiguous role for psychiatry, and for Uganda's growing contingent of AMOs. It reminds us that psychiatry was not a unified force operating in the service of empire.

DISSENT IN 1940S BUGANDA

Samwiri Wamala became *Katikiro* in 1941 in the wake of the *Nnamasole* (Queen Mother) affair, a controversy surrounding her proposed remarriage, and against a backdrop of increasing political, economic and social tension in Buganda.[47] In the years following the Second World War, farmers complained of poor wages, diminished by post-war inflation, colonial cotton regulations and exploitative middlemen.[48] Bataka protesters such as Jemusi Miti and Ssemakula Mulumba also developed populist critiques of Buganda's hierarchy and relationship to colonial power, constructing, as Carol Summers has argued, 'a new sort of citizenship grounded in local concerns over land, graves, and inheritance'.[49] According to David Apter, Wamala was 'the first *Katikiro* to reckon with public opinion', harnessing widespread fear and distrust of missionaries and administrators in his attempt to achieve political reform.[50] His attempt to prevent the colonial administration from forcing the

Lukiiko (Buganda Parliament) to pass legislation that would allow the *Kabaka* (King of Buganda) to acquire land for public use, for example, saw Wamala not only advising the colonial Resident of Uganda that the Bill would be exceedingly unpopular, but also directing public outcry towards his political rivals. While he was by no means the most outspoken of the Ganda activists of the 1940s, his prominent position in the *Lukiiko* and his criticisms of the colonial government's acquisition of land at Mulago (for Mulago Hospital) and Makerere (for Makerere College) placed him at the centre of British attention and concern.[51]

The decision to summon Wamala to a formal medical board was taken in the face of these strained relations between Buganda and the colonial government. Yet it does not appear to have been without some medical justification. In May–June 1944, Wamala had consulted two AMOs—Erifazi Mukibi-Mwanjale and Samuel B. K. Mukasa, Wamala's son-in-law—about a number of physical and mental complaints.[52] By 1944, Mukibi-Mwanjale, a member of the Lugave (pangolin) clan that comprised Wamala's main political support base, was a well-established surgeon at Mulago Hospital.[53] According to Mukibi-Mwanjale some months later, Wamala had exhibited signs of overwork and had improved following a period of 'rest, suggestion, reassurance talks about his hidden fears, [and] regulation of his diet with extra vitamins'.[54] He also admitted, however, to giving Wamala a course of tryparsamide, a treatment used in cases of neurosyphilis.[55]

It was the possibility of neurosyphilis that the medical board was most interested in when it met at Mulago Hospital at the end of October 1944. Formally organised by the Resident of Buganda, and supposedly without the knowledge of the *Lukiiko*, the medical board consisted of H. C. Trowell, who at the time was in charge of admissions to Mulago Mental Hospital, as well as A. W. Williams, Physician and later Medical Superintendent of Mulago Hospital, and an AMO from Buganda, Sebastiane B. Kyewalyanga.[56] Members of the Buganda Government were not obliged to undergo routine medical examinations, but they could be summoned to attend a government medical board if suspicion of serious ill-health arose. In an example that shows how medical missionaries were willing to intrude in local politics, CMS mission doctor Albert Cook stressed in 1926 that he considered it his 'duty' not just as a doctor but as a British subject to inform the colonial administration that his patient, *Katikiro* Apollo Kagwa, was suffering from 'alarmingly high blood pressure', something that Kagwa later claimed had been a deliberate attempt to get him removed from office.[57] In Wamala's case, it is unclear if Mukibi-Mwanjale or Mukasa had passed on their concerns or if the information had reached colonial officials through other channels. Mukibi-Mwanjale was certainly (and unsurprisingly) keen to disassociate himself from the findings of the medical board when they were reported at the beginning of November. His medical testimony, he claimed, had been misinterpreted, and 'so framed as to indicate to any reader that my patient had no other symptoms but mental, and no other treatment but tryparsamide'.[58]

If Mukibi-Mwanjale was unhappy with the board's findings, Kyewalyanga, the board's only AMO, also found himself in an uncomfortable position. The board had failed to find conclusive evidence that Wamala was suffering from neurosyphilis: he had refused a lumbar puncture, something 'essential in the diagnosis of neuro-syphilis', and the board had found 'little outside information concerning the mental symptoms from those in close contact with the patient', without which it was near 'impossible to give a decision concerning [the] presence of mental disease'.[59] Following a brief physical examination, Trowell and Williams were ready to conclude that it was highly likely that Wamala was suffering from neurosyphilis. Kyewalyanga, on the other hand, was more cautious. On his request, the diagnosis of neurosyphilis was removed from the board's findings, and the final statement reworded to conclude that there was 'a serious mental disorder and that the presence of neuro-syphilis cannot be excluded'. Given this finding, the board recommended that Wamala be removed from office for a period of twelve months.[60]

In this instance, psychiatry was no unproblematic, conspiratorial 'tool of empire' for either the European or the African doctors. Even if Wamala's actions had given the British grounds to distrust him, all of the doctors involved agreed that Wamala was suffering from (or had suffered from) mental ill-health, however defined. In a note attached to the bottom of the medical board's report, Trowell and Williams urged Mukibi-Mwanjale and Mukasa to continue the treatment for neurosyphilis, 'as in our opinion the disease is probably there'.[61] Where the doctors diverged was in their view of what function the medical board could serve—the AMOs were particularly sensitive to the political and moral implications of a diagnosis of degenerative venereal disease.[62] Indeed, the whole episode was characterised by political and professional tensions: between Mukibi-Mwanjale and the medical board; between Wamala and the medical board; and between Kyewalyanga and his European colleagues.

These tensions were indicative of wider socio-economic and political discontent that was to prompt widespread disturbances in 1945 and
1949. The strikes and riots of January 1945 were primarily a result of
wage grievances following the hardships of the Second World War, and
saw workers from nearly every government institution walk out and
demand higher wages.[63] At Mulago Hospital, large numbers of subordinate staff joined the strike, and on the second day, strikers entered the
wards with sticks in an attempt to force the remaining African staff to
leave.[64] In the weeks following the strikes, the education system came
under attack from those who felt that the strike demonstrated how easily
hospital workers 'could just chuck up their jobs and cause suffering to
their own people'.[65]

While African doctors were not exempt from scrutiny, there is little
evidence to suggest that they left their positions on the wards. According
to E. Wilson, Physician at Mulago Hospital, Mukibi-Mwanjale 'stood
and appealed to the strikers not to drive away those who were caring for
their own people - we had several badly injured rioters on that ward'.[66]
Indicating something of the position of the mental hospital in the mind
of the public, one 'Onlooker' even jumped to the defence of the staff at
Mulago Hospital by pointing out how: 'the Strike was confined to the
menial staff, cooks, dhobies, sweepers, and the majority of the attendants
in the Mental Section of the Hospital. None of the ward nursing staff or
African doctors was absent from work, and all carried out their duties in
circumstances of great difficulty despite intimidating threats'.[67]

In an attempt to analyse the disturbances, the colonial government
focused on the political, rather than the economic causes, stressing 'the
factional ambitions of a limited number of politicians in Buganda'.[68]
Wamala again came under the spotlight, the strikes having been used
by Wamala's supporters to secure his arch rival's dismissal in case he was
promoted to *Katikiro* in Wamala's absence.[69] Forced to resign at the end
of February, Wamala was promptly deported to Hoima along with four
others suspected of inciting trouble.[70] The severity with which the colonial government pursued Wamala was not lost on at least one observer,
who questioned how the British could deport a man found to be mentally unwell to a place of 'ill treatment'.[71] Deportation, it appears, was a
more straightforward way of dealing with suspected troublemakers than
formal certification and confinement in a mental hospital.

If the relationship between psychiatry and colonial rule was made
problematic by the involvement of AMOs in medical examinations,

it was further complicated by the suspicion that fell on staff at Mulago Hospital following the 1945 disturbances. Mukibi-Mwanjale, for example, was accused of harbouring sympathies towards the activists and was subsequently transferred to the remote station of Moyo where, according to Iliffe, 'he could not practise surgery, was kept under surveillance, suffered a mental breakdown, retired, and never recovered'.[72] Bosa was also reported as being 'anti-European' in confidential reports submitted to the Medical Department, and his progress closely monitored until well into the 1950s.

Particular attention was paid to Bosa during the summer of 1949, when he was arrested in connection with further disturbances that spread across Buganda in April 1949. Bosa had provided a medical certificate to a man calling himself Yusufu Musoke, which showed he had been in hospital suffering from dysentery for the duration of the disturbances.[73] According to Bosa, while he was working in the outpatient department at Mulago Hospital in June, a young man approached him with an old Medical Form 5 (record of patient treatment). The form was 'wrinkled and partially torn', and the accompanying Medical Certificate, due to having been accidentally 'washed in his trouser pocket', 'was now illegible and therefore not acceptable by his employer who threatened to cut his pay'.[74] Bosa agreed to rewrite and sign the certificate, 'which at the time I thought was genuine and therefore I did not think of checking up the number in the Register....Apparently this man knew me very well although I did not know him at the time'.[75] 'From that time I forgot everything about the affair', Bosa added, 'until I was approached by a Police Officer on 13th August, and I was only then made to understand that that man had come to me with a false certificate, and under a false name; and that he had subsequently attempted to use my signed Medical Certificate to cover another person under charge of a criminal offence'.[76]

Bosa was arrested on charges of false certification and suspended from duty. The evidence was hardly in his favour: the certificate Bosa had provided had been used as an alibi by a man accused of setting fire to the house of a county chief, and the man who had approached Bosa for the medical certificate, whose real name was Petero Nsubuga, was an employee of the mental hospital.[77] In his interview with the police, Bosa admitted wrongly certifying sickness, but claimed that it was due to negligence on his part rather than any conspiracy to subvert the course of justice.[78] Bosa was acquitted, but faced a disciplinary interview with DMS Henry S. de Boer before he was allowed to return to work. Recounting his version of events to de Boer, Bosa observed that his case was only serious because of its 'political connections'—he could see 'No other reason except general need for accuracy'.[79] Indeed, as Bosa was likely aware, the political sympathies of AMOs from across Mulago Hospital again came under suspicion in the months following the disturbances.[80] However much responsibility was being devolved to AMOs, they were still firmly located within the rigid structures of a paternalist colonial hierarchy and were by no means exempt from scrutiny during political troubles.

Bosa was found guilty of negligence and narrowly avoided losing his job, but was allowed to remain at Mulago Mental Hospital. His actions during the 1940s, like those of his colleagues in the Wamala case, belie any straightforward relationship between psychiatry and politics at the end of empire. Was Bosa complicit in Nsubuga's attempt to avoid arrest, using his position at Mulago to undermine the state? Bosa's superiors certainly continued to distrust him, regarding him throughout the 1950s as an 'excellent clinician', yet one who was not above suspicion politically or ethically. Alternatively, was this incompetence, or a disregard for rules and authority? Bosa found himself in trouble with the law again in 1954, having failed to keep a proper register of cocaine hydrochloride as required under the Poisons and Dangerous Drugs Ordinance.[81] He was reprimanded and fined under the Ordinance, but again escaped dismissal. If anything is clear, it is that Bosa had made himself essential to psychiatry, holding onto his job despite repeated reprimands by medical boards and other superiors, as well as ongoing suspicion about his motivation. This uneasy relationship with hierarchy did not go away as the newly independent Ministry of Health took over responsibility for psychiatry in 1962.

BOSA AND HIERARCHIES OF POWER

Bosa returned to Uganda from postgraduate study at the Maudsley Hospital in January 1958 and, following Tewfik's resignation later that year, was made Acting Superintendent of Mulago and Butabika Mental Hospitals. As a temporary position while a replacement for Tewfik could be found, it gave him first-hand experience of managing a full clinical and administrative workload, as well as the challenges facing African doctors within a rapidly Africanising administration. While Bosa appears to have been popular and generally respected by the European nursing staff at the mental hospitals, there were a number of 'more awkward officers' who refused to work beneath him.[82] Responsibility for this was something that the colonial Medical Department placed firmly on Bosa. Rather than this being a question of racism, Bosa reportedly did not have a 'strong enough personality', lacking confidence, being too sensitive, and avoiding administration in favour of clinical work.[83] He was also unwilling to facilitate research, whether due to a desire to protect patients who were not capable of giving consent, or because he had other priorities. In 1959, for example, it was suggested that Bosa had attempted to sabotage a medical survey of tuberculosis conducted on mental patients by G. Murray Short by 'losing' a series of X-rays and generally being 'uncooperative'.[84] These views shaped official assessments about Bosa's ability to successfully manage mental hospital staff in the long term. While they acknowledged that Bosa was working in a 'difficult position' and showed great skill with patients, in 1960, the Medical Department decided to appoint an Australian expatriate psychiatrist, T. W. Murray as Superintendent of Mental Hospitals.[85]

On the award of the DPM in 1961, Bosa was made a consultant psychiatrist. Emboldened by the promotion, Bosa started to send suggestions for the reform of mental health services to senior administrative officials, including Kadama, Chief Medical Officer of the Ministry of Health in 1962, and Permanent Secretary from 1963. Among these were calls for the introduction of a Registered Mental Nurses course, more psychiatric training for African doctors and the expansion of psychiatric wards at up-country hospitals. Ministry of Health officials refused to include Bosa in discussions about the future of medical services, however.[86] In their opinion, Bosa was breaking the chain of command by coming directly to them—he was to address all his concerns to Murray for consideration.[87] Yet they were also annoyed that Bosa had 'committed his ideas to paper before we made a comparable move on our side'.[88] Jealous of their new power as policymakers, they did not want to be seen to be taking advice from a doctor who was not aware of his position in the hierarchy, even if he was Ugandan.

By 1964, Murray and Bosa shared a huge workload, including clinical work at Butabika Hospital and Mulago Hospital Mental Health Clinic, the teaching of undergraduate medical students at Makerere University College, court work and the management of up-country psychiatric wards in Soroti and Mbarara. When Murray took his overseas leave in September 1964, he was requested to 'step aside' to make way for Bosa to become Superintendent of Mental Hospitals.[89] On Murray's return,

Bosa stayed on as Superintendent, and the division of clinical duties between the two was reversed, with Bosa taking on a greater part of the administration. The relationship between the two remained ill-defined, however. Murray was given a new role as 'Adviser', a title he held until his departure in 1966, but this served only to complicate matters: Was he to be an adviser to Bosa, or an independent adviser to the Ministry of Health? As Bosa complained: 'This is a new situation which has not existed here before. One cannot say that Dr. Murray and myself are just reversing the relationship that existed before Dr. Murray went on leave in September 1964. Then I was subordinate to him and could not make direct contact with [the] Ministry of Health' except via Murray, as Medical Superintendent.[90] When an attempt was made to clarify the relationship, again the Ministry of Health remained vague in its response: 'You will see from these letters that you are the substantive Medical Superintendent and that Dr. Murray is a consultant psychiatrist. He will carry on with his normal duties and may advise you if you so wish, he may of course sign correspondence on your behalf but any personal letters written to me by Dr. Murray should be sent' through Bosa, if they refer to official matters.[91]

It was only with Murray's resignation in April 1966 that the ambiguity in the hierarchy at Butabika Hospital was resolved. By that point, however, the Ministry of Health had already demonstrated that it was no more willing to listen to Bosa's petitions for the improvement of psychiatric services than it had been to Murray or any previous psychiatrist. The neglect of psychiatry by the Ministry of Health prompted a clearly frustrated Bosa to protest in October 1965 that the 'work-output which is being demanded from the small number of doctors is ridiculously fantastic. I have often put in a warning that there is such a thing as "demanding too much out of too few for too long"'.[92] The problem was that:

The Ministry have entirely refused to awaken to the modern concept that Psychiatry is medicine; - a type of medicine that is difficult, exacting and very time-consuming. They have refused to appreciate that Butabika Hospital is practically the only and total psychiatric service for the whole of Uganda (you can more or less discount the ridiculous so-called psychiatric units in the Eastern and Western Regions; I always regard them as an insult to psychiatry), and that as such, the medical team at Butabika has to put in a terrific amount of hard work to keep pace with the very high admission rate in the already overcrowded Wards. Can any doctor carry on at this rate indefinitely? No Sir. In the long run the efficiency must drop, and that may be followed by disasterous [sic.] consequences. THIS HAS STARTED TO HAPPEN HERE.[93]

Just because a Ugandan was in charge of mental health services, it did not mean that the financial or professional support required to develop psychiatry was more forthcoming. Exhausted by the administrative workload, Bosa resigned as Superintendent at the end of 1965, but continued to work as a consultant psychiatrist at Mulago and Butabika. J. Bulwanyi, a non-specialist Senior Medical Officer and Superintendent of Fort Portal Hospital, was chosen as the new Superintendent of Mental Hospitals, allowing Bosa to commit himself more fully to his clinical duties.[94] In the longer term, the indifference of the government towards psychiatry was reinforced by the realisation that Makerere University College were allocating funds for a Department of Psychiatry within Makerere Medical School. In response to one of Bosa's petitions in 1964, a senior official within the Ministry of Health noted that 'We are lucky that Makerere has now decided to create a Chair of Psychiatry… [as]…the whole question of psychiatry will be adequately handled'.[95] Not only would the department result in more funding and specialist personnel for Butabika and the mental health unit at Mulago Hospital, but responsibility for the development of mental health services would no longer be solely in their hands.

THE DEPARTMENT OF PSYCHIATRY

When the question of psychiatry was first considered by the Faculty Board of Makerere Medical School in 1959, A. W. Williams and colleagues gave three main reasons for the urgency of its development as an academic subject. First, in practical terms, the colonial administration had encountered difficulties in recruiting a psychiatrist to replace Tewfik at Mulago and Butabika Mental Hospitals following his resignation in 1958. In the context of a rapidly decolonising empire, positions within the Colonial Medical Service no longer carried the prestige or opportunities for career progression. As a part-time lecturer for the Medical School, Tewfik had provided courses on mental illness and psychology to first and third clinical year students yet now, despite new recognition of the importance of 'the psychological factors in health and disease, we have no one with the time or qualifications to give to this essential part of the medical course'.[96] Second, there was 'accumulated evidence' from the Student Health Service at Makerere University College on the social and personal stresses facing students. While the Faculty Board noted that there was nothing new in this, or indeed unique to African students, 'it has a specially urgent importance in East Africa where the potential output of graduates is so small in relation to the need, and the social and personal stresses to which this small population of educated adolescents is subjected are correspondingly greater'.[97] Finally, the Board stressed their conviction 'that because of language difficulties and cultural attitudes psychiatry among Africans will best be practised by Africans'.[98] For this, the Board stressed that Makerere had 'a special responsibility to undertake a study of the psychological implications of higher education in East Africa', and that an understanding of the 'conditions in which [the] postgraduate training of African psychiatrists to work in Africa can be undertaken are needed'.[99] Makerere had a unique status in East Africa as the premier institution for education and research and had close ties with the East African Institute of Social Research (EAISR) under Audrey Richards, making it an ideal setting for psychiatric education and research.

In looking for advice, Makerere Medical School turned to the Nuffield Foundation's visiting consultant scheme. Makerere had already benefited from the scheme on numerous occasions since the late 1940s, though none had been psychiatrists.[100] The application revealed a Faculty Board that was keen to proceed with the development of psychiatry as an academic subject, but which was concerned that due to the financial implications, it would 'have to face a rigorous examination by the East African Governments', so requiring expertise to ensure a strong case for support.[101] While Makerere was a semi-autonomous institution, control over administrative and financial decisions was not always clear, particularly within medicine, where Mulago Hospital was both a government hospital and a university teaching institution. Makerere sought a consultant for a three-month visit, who would be able to provide advice on appointments, recruitment, the relationship of staff with the Education and Social Anthropology departments, as well as the Student Health Service, the relationship of the teaching department to the mental hospital, priorities for research, and the training of Africans in psychiatry.[102] The application was successful, and a few months later, Davies, of the Maudsley Hospital, arrived for an eight-week tour.

Echoing wider sentiments within Africa about the unique potential of African psychiatrists, Davies noted that 'Psychiatry is the one branch of medicine in which the African doctor starts with an advantage over his expatriate colleague by reason of his greater knowledge of local language and custom'.[103] The current curriculum, however, involved only minimal instruction in psychiatry which, combined with short-term placements in the under-funded and overcrowded mental hospital, gave 'no hope for the recruitment of Makerere graduates to this specialty, and this will nullify any attempt to improve the government services substantially'.[104] Davies suggested the creation of a Department of Psychiatry at Makerere Medical School, with a Professorial Chair, to be organised along English lines.[105] In addition to the chair, the department would require two lecturers, two house officers, one psychiatric social worker, one clinical psychologist, an occupational therapist, nursing staff and a secretarial assistant.[106] A unit focused on rehabilitation would also be required, away from Butabika Hospital, which was still predominantly engaged in the long-term care of patients, and included a wing for criminal lunatics. As Davies noted, 'If prestige factors are important, and if psychiatry is to take its place alongside medicine and surgery as a major branch of medicine in this country then the medical student must be introduced to it in a place freed from the aura of prisons'.[107] A new unit at Mulago Hospital was required, with teaching space and a ward for 30–40 patients, to be selected according to the teaching and research needs of the professor. There was little comment on how the curriculum could be made relevant to East Africa, however. Instead, Davies drew on recent articles from *The Lancet*, reports of the Royal College of Physicians and recommendations of the GMC. The only indication that the reach of psychiatry in Uganda differed from that in the UK was Davies' reminder that the selection of doctors for specialist training and the local recruitment of student mental nurses should be done 'with an eye to the language problem'.[108]

Makerere University College received Davies' report with interest, and in 1960, the principal formed an internal committee to advise on how Davies' recommendations might be implemented.[109] Despite the enthusiasm of the committee to implement Davies' plan, however, neither Makerere University College nor the colonial government felt they could commit to funding a Department of Psychiatry.[110] Not only was medical expansion in general constrained by finances, but psychiatry remained a low priority in a country where government expenditure

was directed towards revenue producing activities and general education.[111] Instead, the committee turned to external funding sources, considering the suitability of joint Makerere-Government applications to a
range of international bodies, including the Ford Foundation and the
US International Cooperation Administration (ICA).[112] Funding bodies already supported teaching at Makerere Medical School—UNICEF
most recently providing for a Foundation Chair of Paediatrics—but in
the early 1960s there was little international interest in the promotion
of psychiatry in Africa, and with only limited support from the Ministry
of Health, it was a further six years before Makerere was able to allocate
funds.[113]

The Department of Psychiatry at Makerere Medical School opened in
March 1966 with the arrival of the Foundation Professor of Psychiatry.
Born in Scotland, G. Allen German had been advised to apply for the
position by Sir Aubrey Lewis while working as a Senior Psychiatric
Registrar at the Maudsley Hospital.[114] A few weeks after German's
arrival, Murray left the country, leaving German and Bosa as the only
psychiatrists in Uganda. Looking to fill this government vacancy with
someone who would be keen to support his plans for development,
German wrote to his brother-in-law, James F. Wood, a Senior Registrar
at the Ross Clinic, Aberdeen, inviting him to join him in Uganda. Wood
accepted, arriving at Butabika Hospital as a government consultant psychiatrist a few months later. From the start of his professorship, German
was able to wield considerable influence over appointments like that of
Wood, as well as clinical practice at Ward 16 (the mental health ward at
Mulago Hospital), Mulago Hospital Mental Health Clinic (an outpatient
department that had opened in 1964) and Butabika Hospital.[115] While
German was technically employed by Makerere University College,
on his arrival he became the de facto head of mental health services in
Uganda.

One of the key features of the new Department of Psychiatry was the
cooperation it demanded between university and government. In the
original plans for the department, it was intended that the department
and outpatient psychiatric unit at Mulago Hospital 'should be comple-
mentary to that of the Butabika hospital....Butabika psychiatrists should
be appointed visiting consultants at the Mulago Unit, and the professor and lecturer at Butabika Hospital'.[116] The department and unit at
Mulago Hospital would mark the start of a new, 'modern' era of mental

health care, providing a space for the training of African doctors as well as psychiatric nurses, psychiatric social workers and occupational therapists.[117] This collaboration, of course, had financial implications—salaries, equipment and travelling expenses all required negotiation—but it also meant that the staff available for clinical, teaching and forensic work was immediately increased: as was usual practice at Mulago Hospital, all government psychiatrists were appointed as honorary lecturers at Makerere University College, and the academic psychiatrists were consultants in government service.[118] In contrast to other specialisms, this collaboration appears to have caused little tension or resentment on either side.[119] Indeed, the fierce negotiations between university and government over the duties of other staff at Mulago Hospital during the 1960s, with its widespread 'ill-feeling', appear to have passed the psychiatrists by. This did not, however, prevent personality clashes between individual psychiatrists. The relationship between Bosa and Bulwanyi, for example, was plagued by constant personal disagreements, dividing staff at Butabika Hospital and eventually requiring Ministry of Health intervention.[120] Responsibility for teaching and clinical work also remained ill-defined, with teaching requirements not written into contracts until the end of the decade.[121]

Between 1966 and 1969, teaching provision in psychiatry at undergraduate level expanded from twenty hours to three hundred, more than that in most medical schools in the UK.[122] Such was the extent of the changes that on a return visit in 1969 Davies remarked on how impressed he was by the amount of time devoted to psychiatry, as well as to the behavioural sciences more generally, something 'in line with the most advanced views in medical education'.[123] Teaching consisted of clerking on inpatients and outpatients, as well as lectures and small group seminars designed to prepare doctors to have 'sufficient grounding in Psychiatry to be capable of providing basic psychiatric care in district hospitals and up-country areas' not just in Uganda but across East Africa.[124] While the syllabus broadly followed that of medical schools in the UK, the lecturers were aware of the need to make teaching locally relevant. John H. Orley, an anthropologist and psychiatrist attached to the Department of Psychiatry, 1966–1968 and 1971–1973, gave occasional lectures on his research on mental illness and epilepsy among the Ganda. Wood, moreover, took organic causes of mental illness as one of his subjects, something he felt was key to reducing the high number of unnecessary referrals to the mental health clinic.[125] His lectures on the topic included the definitions, features and causes of mental confusion and acute brain syndromes, as well as the steps involved in a basic examination.[126]

While the teaching at undergraduate level aimed primarily at producing general practitioners who had a good understanding of how to recognise and manage mental illness, these lecturers also hoped to encourage African medical practitioners to specialise in psychiatry. Those wishing to attain an MMed, introduced at Makerere Medical School in 1968, were required to complete a three-month attachment to Butabika Hospital.[127] By 1971, the one-year course of instruction for the Diploma in Public Health (DPH), a requirement for doctors aspiring to be a Medical Officer of Health or to any senior administrative post in the Ministry of Health, also included a full week of thirty-seven hours (practical and theoretical) in mental health.[128] These training schemes were supported by grants from international bodies, which allowed the Department of Psychiatry to appoint new lecturers and researchers. Orley, whose interest in East Africa had been developed by E. E. Evans-Pritchard and John Beattie at the University of Oxford, was funded during his first two years in Uganda by a Nuffield Foundation research grant.[129] The Norwegian aid agency, NORAD, sponsored the secondment of Arvid Aas, a Professor of Clinical Psychology at the University of Oslo, to Makerere University College for a period of two years.[130] The World Health Organization (WHO), too, provided financial support for a lecturer in psychiatry, a position that was awarded to H. G. Egdell, a specialist in child psychiatry, in 1968.[131]

Despite these efforts, the number of African doctors specialising in psychiatry remained low throughout the 1960s. Just as Bosa had been transferred to Mulago Mental Hospital in 1948, African doctors were placed at Butabika Hospital, with few opting to pursue it independently. Once attached to Butabika Hospital, graduates were assessed for their suitability for further training, and if interested might then be allowed to pursue a formal postgraduate qualification. E. B. Ssekabembe, who had qualified as a doctor in India, had been attached to Butabika Hospital since 1964 at least and by 1966 was in London preparing for the DPM.[132] Wilson Acuda, too, graduated from Makerere Medical School in 1970. His initial placement at Butabika Hospital for a period of one year was not of his choosing, but he 'fell in love with Psychiatry within a few weeks' and was determined to specialise in it. After six months at

Butabika Hospital, he was offered a scholarship by the British Council to study at the Maudsley Hospital from April 1972, an opportunity that he accepted.[133]

The expansion of training at postgraduate level was assisted by the creation in 1966 of three Senior House Officer (SHO) positions in psychiatry. These were designed for doctors who had not undertaken formal training in psychiatry but who had considerable experience in psychiatric practice.[134] A. T. Kikwanguyira, who had been attached to Butabika Hospital since 1966 at least, was raised to one of these positions, allowing for the recognition of his experience with the mentally ill.[135] Intending to make full use of these new positions, German noted in 1967 that '[i]t is envisaged that S.H.O.s will train on an in-service basis and that, for the moment, they will continue to proceed to London to take their Diploma in Psychological Medicine. A series of lectures at postgraduate level has been given over the past session and the present S.H.O. is due to take the first part of the D.P.M. in London in May 1967'.[136] This SHO was Joseph Muhangi, who on his return to Uganda worked as a Special Grade Medical Officer (Psychiatry) before being appointed as a lecturer in the Department of Psychiatry in November 1969.[137] Another SHO, A. M. Kitumba followed a few years later, completing the MRCPsych in London in 1972.[138]

In the years following the opening of the Department of Psychiatry in March 1966, Uganda saw an increase in the number of expatriate psychiatrists from one to six by 1969 (including one psychiatric social worker). With formal and informal programmes designed to train African doctors, too, the number of African psychiatrists also rose from one to three.[139] When Davies returned to Uganda in 1969 to re-evaluate the state of psychiatry, he was particularly impressed by the speed of change and reported finding a united group of psychiatrists, led by German, but with posts filled evenly between Ugandans and expatriates.[140] This divide between expatriates and Ugandans broadly reflected that at Makerere Medical School more generally, where by 1971, 38% of staff was Ugandan. While this was better than the situation in 1965, when only 11% of the academic staff was Ugandan, it was still nowhere near that of the university administration, where 81% of staff was Ugandan.[141] 'Despite political pressure to "Africanize" as rapidly as possible', W. D. Foster has noted, 'the senior Ugandan members of the college were as unwilling as anyone to see' people they regarded as 'unsuitable men appointed to chairs merely because they were Ugandans'.[142]

CONCLUSION

It is perhaps ironic that the body of research on detribalisation, developed by the East African School of Psychiatry and Psychology, and premised on assumptions of racial and cultural difference, had provided the first arguments for the training of Africans in psychiatry. Summing up the expectations for this new generation of doctors, H. J. Simons, of the University of Cape Town, noted that in East Africa, African psychiatrists 'would combine, as few other practitioners can do, the required knowledge of medicine and psychiatry with an intimate knowledge of the people's physiognomy, language, and traits'.[143] In practice, as I explore further in subsequent chapters, the idea that Africans might have natural cultural 'insight' into their patients' fears and anxieties was deeply flawed, and overlooked the vast cultural, social and linguistic gap that also existed between Western-trained African doctors and many of their patients. Before the 1960s, however, it received little overt criticism from Ugandan doctors. In the context of professionalisation and attempts to secure better working conditions, pay and status within the colonial medical hierarchy, such arguments served an important political purpose.

While concerns about the need to prepare for psychiatry to respond to the challenges and pressures of rapid social and political change were expressed across Eastern and Southern Africa, it was Uganda that claimed a 'special responsibility' to act. Enacted as part of broader policies of 'Africanisation' at the end of empire, the Africanisation of psychiatry encompassed the secondment of African doctors to Mulago Mental Hospital (and later Butabika) for short-term placements, opportunities for doctors such as Bosa to undertake postgraduate study in the UK, and the eventual elevation of Bosa to Medical Superintendent. Taking up the call to promote psychiatry as a field of study and research, Makerere University College also led a rapid expansion of clinical and academic psychiatry during the 1960s and early 1970s. The influx of expatriate psychiatrists that this entailed was, nevertheless, at odds with the processes of Africanisation, and would have implications for the decolonisation of psychiatry, and who had a say. One of the ways Makerere navigated this was to increase the turnover of expatriate staff, appointing new lecturers on contracts of up to six years rather than on a permanent basis.[144] Yet it was not without its limitations, particularly for psychiatry, where communication was central. As F. J. Bennett noted in 1965, the 'disadvantages of employing foreigners on short contracts in a country with at least 25 language groups can be imagined'.[145]

The increase in the number of doctors trained in psychiatry may have had limited practical effect on the willingness of government administrators to provide additional resources for psychiatry, but it is nevertheless important for our understanding of the role and power of psychiatry at the end of empire. The inclusion of African doctors within the formal structures and institutions of colonial psychiatry remind us that psychiatry was no straightforward tool of 'social control' wielded by the colonial government. African doctors were working in contexts rich in actors and politics of their own, with psychiatry operating in spaces that show a much more complex relationship to colonial power than that of 'tool of empire'. The potential use of psychiatry to subvert colonial authority during political dissent in Buganda during the 1940s, for example, provides an important counterpoint to narratives of the mobilisation of psychiatry in the service of empire during the years of decolonisation. Indeed, it proved impossible to separate psychiatry from politics that extended beyond the strictly 'imperial'. In a letter to Davies in 1960, Bosa relayed fears that if he were to leave the relative safety of government service he doubted being able to 'survive very long in the present "political" climate'.[146] Traders in Wandegeya market had refused to sell to him because 'they did not like my attitude towards the trade boycott campaign, and because my children rode on the bus to and from school'.[147] If he were to open a private clinic and did not follow what he regarded as the ridiculous demands of the Ganda elite, he speculated that he 'would probably end up in Kololo Mortuary with multiple bullet holes from a "made in Masaka" rifle. I doubt whether my children would like that'.[148] Psychiatry may have been neglected and underdeveloped as a medical discipline, but it did not mean that psychiatrists occupied a neutral political space. Local and national politics would only become more relevant for psychiatry in the years following Independence.

NOTES

1. D. Mackay, 'A Background for African Psychiatry', *East African Medical Journal* 25(1) (1948), p. 4.
2. Ibid., p. 2.
3. Ibid., p. 3.
4. Ibid., p. 2.
5. 'Editorial', *East African Medical Journal* 25(1) (1948), p. 1.
6. H. C. Trowell, as cited in J. Iliffe, *East African Doctors: A History of the Modern Profession* (Kampala, 2002), pp. 45–46.
7. Iliffe, *East African Doctors*, p. 60. See also: M. Lyons, 'The Power to Heal: African Medical Auxiliaries in Colonial Belgian Congo and Uganda', in D. Engels and S. Marks, eds., *Contesting Colonial Hegemony: State and Society in Africa and India* (London, 1994).
8. Uganda Protectorate, *Annual Report of the Medical Department for the Year Ended 31 December, 1937* (Entebbe, 1938), p. 6.
9. Eria M. Babumba, 'An African Patient', *East African Medical Journal* 31(8) (1954), p. 373.
10. Uganda Ministry of Health Archives (UMOHA) PH/ASC/46 (Box 29) (Makerere Medical Graduates Association), f. 9, 'A discussion between the Hon'ble the Director of Medical Services and the Makerere Medical Graduates Associations' Delegation', 1950.
11. H. C. Trowell, 'Training Medical Practitioners', *East African Medical Journal* 33(7) (1956), p. 257.
12. Trowell, 'Training Medical Practitioners', p. 257.
13. As cited in F. Heinlein, *British Government Policy and Decolonisation 1945–1963: Scrutinising the Official Mind* (London, 2002), p. 25.
14. Iliffe, *East African Doctors*, pp. 118–120.
15. Heinlein, *British Government Policy*, p. 25.
16. J. L. Crammer, 'Training and Education in British Psychiatry 1770–1970', in H. Freeman and G. Berrios, eds., *150 Years of British Psychiatry* (London, 1996), pp. 221–228.
17. The National Archives, Kew, United Kingdom (TNA) BW 90/16 (East Africa—Medical School Mulago), memo by E. G. Holmes, Makerere College, 'Makerere College Medical School and Mulago Hospital—An Appreciation of the Present Situation', 24 November 1947, pp. 2–3; *Report of the Council to the Assembly for the Year 1946* (Kampala, 1947), p. 11.
18. Bodleian Library, University of Oxford (BOD) Mss.Afr.s.1589 (Baty Papers), 'Hospital Routine', ff. 2–3, 'Instructions on routine to be carried out by A.M.O. attached to Mental Hospital, 28 March 1946'.
19. Crammer, 'Training and Education in British Psychiatry'; Trowell, 'Training Medical Practitioners', p. 255.

20. Uganda Protectorate, *Annual Report of the Medical Department for the Year Ended 31st December, 1938* (Entebbe, 1939), pp. 67–68.
21. TNA CO 536/199/7 (Mental Treatment Legislation), 'Legal Report on an Ordinance entitled "The Mental Treatment Ordinance, 1938"', p. 2.
22. J. E. Goldthorpe, *An African Elite: Makerere College Students 1922– 1960* (Nairobi, 1965), p. 46; F. G. Sembeguya, 'The Growth of an Indigenous Medical Profession', *East African Medical Journal* 41(2) (1964), p. 40.
23. UMOHA C90/ACR (Bosa Stephen B—Consult. Psychiat.), f. 35, letter from W. A. Wilson to G. Campbell Young, 17 February 1953.
24. Uganda National Archives (UNA) C1304 (Benjamin Kagwa).
25. B. H. Kagwa, *A Ugandan: Defiant and Triumphant* (Hicksville, 1978), p. 23.
26. TNA CO 536/207/11 (Kagwa B—Native Student).
27. TNA CO 536/207/11, f. 4, extract from letter from Dr. Kauntze to Dr. O'Brien, 9 March 1940.
28. TNA CO 536/207/11, f. 1, letter from J. E. W. Flood to A. J. R. O'Brien, 27 December 1939, pp. 4–5.
29. TNA CO 536/207/11, f. 5, 'Negro Physician from Central Africa', *St. Louis Post-Dispatch*, 27 August 1940; Kagwa, *A Ugandan*, p. 113.
30. Kagwa, *A Ugandan*, p. 91.
31. Kagwa, *A Ugandan*, p. 105.
32. Kagwa, *A Ugandan*, pp. 114–115; 'Manhattan Central Medical Society— N.Y.C.', *Journal of the National Medical Association* 41(1) (1949), p. 38.
33. UMOHA C90/ACR.
34. BOD Mss.Afr.s.1589, 'Correspondence', ff. J. C. Carothers, 'Report on the existing organisation in Uganda for the care and treatment of persons of unsound mind and the question of the future development of this organisation', 1 February 1943.
35. BOD Mss.Afr.s.1589, 'Correspondence', f. 11, copy of the 'Recommendations of the Mental Hospital Enquiry Committee', 11 February 1942. Complaints about the lack of accommodation for Europeans, for example, had been made in 1941 in UNA D107/12 (Transport of Mental Patients).
36. BOD Mss.Afr.s.1589, 'Correspondence', ff. 15–16, J. C. Carothers, 'Report on the existing organisation in Uganda for the care and treatment of persons of unsound mind and the question of the future development of this organisation', 1 February 1943, p. 4.
37. BOD Mss.Afr.s.1589, 'Correspondence', f. 14, letter from J. P. Mitchell, Medical Superintendent, Mulago, to Director of Medical Services, Entebbe, 30 March 1943.

38. Iliffe, *East African Doctors*, pp. 65–67.
39. UMOHA C90/ACR, f. 1, 'Annual Confidential Report for the Year Ending December 31st 1947'.
40. Iliffe, *East African Doctors*, pp. 99–100.
41. UMOHA C90/ACR, f. 37, letter from E. M. Clark, for Director of Medical Services, to the Specialist Alienist, Mental Hospital, Mulago, 7 July 1955.
42. Iliffe, *East African Doctors*, p. 100.
43. UMOHA C90/ACR, f. 36, letter from G. Campbell Young to the Director of Medical Services, Entebbe, 1 July 1955; Uganda Protectorate, *Annual Report of the Medical Department for the Year Ended 31 December, 1953* (Entebbe, 1954), p. 40; Uganda Protectorate, *Annual Report of the Medical Department for the Year Ended 31 December, 1954* (Entebbe, 1955), p. 54.
44. UMOHA C90/ACR, f. 38, letter from D. L. Davies, Dean, Institute of Psychiatry, to L. A. Mathias, Uganda Students Adviser, London, 28 October 1957.
45. UMOHA C90/ACR, f. 45, letter from D. L. Davies, Dean, Institute of Psychiatry, to L. A. Mathias, Uganda Students Adviser, London, n.d. (likely January 1958).
46. UMOHA C90/ACR, f. 68, letter from K. E. Underwood Ground to Stephen B. Bosa, 8 September 1960; UMOHA, C90/ACR, f. 72, 'Recommendation for Promotion'.
47. F. Mulindwa, 'The Bataka Agitation and Resistance in Colonial Uganda', *Muwazo* 10(3) (2011), pp. 17–18.
48. J. L. Earle, 'Reading Revolution in Late Colonial Buganda', *Journal of Eastern African Studies* 6(3) (2012), pp. 507–508.
49. C. Summers, 'Grandfathers, Grandsons, Morality, and Radical Politics in Late Colonial Buganda', *International Journal of African Historical Studies* 38(5) (2005), p. 427. During the 1940s, the term Bataka came to refer to those who wished to redefine British and Ganda policies and roles. Historically, it had other meanings, notably as a term denoting hereditary clan leaders. For a fuller treatment of political dissent in 1940s Buganda, see especially D. E. Apter, *The Political Kingdom in Uganda: A Study of Bureaucratic Nationalism* (Princeton, NJ: Princeton University Press, 1967), p. 141; F. Mulindwa, 'The *Bataka* Agitation and Resistance in Colonial Uganda', *Muwazo* 10(3) (2011), pp. 12–24; R. Reid, *A History of Modern Uganda* (Cambridge, 2017), pp. 297–311; and G. Thompson, 'Colonialism in Crisis: The Uganda Disturbances of 1945', *African Affairs* 91 (1992), pp. 605–624.
50. Apter, *The Political Kingdom in Uganda*, p. 226.
51. Ibid., pp. 226–227.

52. BOD Mss.Brit.Emp.S.22 G.552 (Anti-slavery Society Papers: Uganda), 'Copy of the Medical Board Report', 30 October 1944.
53. Iliffe, *East African Doctors*, p. 88.
54. BOD Mss.Brit.Emp.S.22 G.552, letter from S. Mukibi Mwanjale, Mulago Hospital, to H. C. Trowell, copy to the Kabaka, and the Director of Medical Services, Entebbe, 9 November 1944.
55. J. D. Hurn, 'The History of General Paralysis of the Insane in Britain, 1830 to 1950' (Unpublished PhD thesis, University of London, 1998), pp. 242–243.
56. BOD Mss.Brit.Emp.S.22 G.552, note by K. B. Maindi, Acting President General, the Uganda Motor Drivers Association Trade Union, attached to a copy of a letter from F. R. Bell to the Resident, Buganda, 24 October 1944.
57. Albert Cook Memorial Library, Makerere University (ACMM), Mengo Hospital Correspondence, letter from A. R. Cook, Mengo Hospital, to Mr. Jarvis, 26 April 1926.
58. BOD Mss.Brit.Emp.S.22 G.552, letter from Mukibi Mwanjale to Trowell, 9 November 1944.
59. BOD Mss.Brit.Emp.S.22 G.552, 'Copy of Medical Board Report', 30 October 1944.
60. Ibid.
61. Ibid.
62. M. W. Tuck, 'Syphilis, Sexuality, and Social Control: A History of Venereal Disease in Colonial Uganda' (Unpublished PhD thesis, Northwestern University, 1997), Ch. 5.
63. Iliffe, *East African Doctors*, p. 89; C. Summers, 'Radical Rudeness: Ugandan Social Critiques in the 1940s', *Journal of Social History* 39(3) (2006), pp. 750–751.
64. Iliffe, *East African Doctors*, p. 89.
65. 'Comment on the Strike', *Uganda Herald*, 21 February 1945, p. 10.
66. E. Wilson, as cited in Iliffe, *East African Doctors*, p. 89.
67. '"Onlooker" on the Strike', *Uganda Herald*, 7 March 1945, p. 4.
68. Thompson, 'Colonialism in Crisis', p. 605.
69. Iliffe, *East African Doctors*, p. 89.
70. House of Commons (HC) Hansard, United Kingdom, Deb 7 March 1945, vol. 408, c2014 (Uganda [Deportation Order]); 'Katikiro Tenders Resignation', *Uganda Herald*, 28 February 1945, p. 5; and 'Om. S. S. Wamala Arrested and Deported', *Uganda Herald*, 7 March 1945, p. 1.
71. BOD Mss.Brit.Emp.S.22 G.552, note by Maindi, 24 October 1944. Wamala was not the only deportee linked to 'ill treatment'. According to Summers, intelligence reports on Festo Kibuka Musoke 'suggested

that by the time he came out of detention after the 1945 strike, he seemed "mentally unbalanced"'. Summers, 'Radical Rudeness', fn. 8.

72. Iliffe, *East African Doctors*, pp. 89–90.

73. UMOHA C90/ACR, letter from R. S. F. Hennessey to Mr. S. B. Bosa, 6 September 1949.

74. UMOHA C90/ACR, letter from S. B. Bosa, Assistant Medical Officer, Mulago, to Director of Medical Services, 5 September 1949.

75. UMOHA C90/ACR, letter from Bosa to Director of Medical Services, 5 September 1949.

76. Ibid.

77. UMOHA C90/ACR, letter from Senior Superintendent of Police, Kampala, to Medical Superintendent, Mulago, 31 August 1949; UMOHA C90/ACR, H. S. de Boer, 'Interview: A.M.O. S.B. Bosa, 6 September 1949'.

78. UMOHA C90/ACR, f. 5, letter from A. W. Williams, Medical Superintendent, Mulago, to Director of Medical Services, 15 August 1949.

79. UMOHA C90/ACR, H. S. de Boer, 'Interview: A.M.O. S.B. Bosa, 6 September 1949'.

80. Iliffe, *East African Doctors*, pp. 90–91.

81. UMOHA C90/ACR, letter from S. B. Bosa to the Registrar, Uganda Medical Board, 30 June 1954.

82. UMOHA C90/ACR, f. 56, 'Stephen B. Bosa, Annual Confidential Report, 1959'.

83. Ibid.; UMOHA, C90/ACR, f. 55, G. I. Tewfik, 'Staff Report—Dr. Bosa'.

84. UMOHA C90/ACR, f. 57, letter from G. Murray Short to C. W. Davies, Director of Medical Services, 18 December 1959.

85. UMOHA C90/ACR, f. 58, 'Stephen B. Bosa, Annual Confidential Report, 1960'.

86. UMOHA C90/ACR, minute 10, no date (likely 1964); UMOHA C90/ACR, minute 8, by S.M.O. (T), 17 February 1964.

87. UMOHA C90/ACR, minute 11, PS/CMO to D.C.M.O., 4 June 1964.

88. UMOHA C90/ACR, minute 8, by S.M.O. (T), 17 February 1964.

89. UMOHA C90/ACR, f. 81, letter from I. S. Kadama to S. B. Bosa, 4 June 1964.

90. UMOHA C90/ACR, f. 91, letter from Stephen Bosa to I. S. Kadama, 27 March 1965.

91. UMOHA C90/ACR, f. 92, letter from I. S. Kadama to S. Bosa, 12 April 1965.

92. UMOHA C90/ACR, f. 94, letter from Stephen Bosa to the Permanent Secretary/Chief Medical Officer, Ministry of Health, 16 October 1965.

93. Ibid.
94. UMOHA GCT.8 (Ministers' Tours [Excluding H.E. The President]), f. 66, 'Medical and Health Services in Ankole and Toro', 17 September 1965, Schedule II.
95. UMOHA C90/ACR, minute 10, n.d., c. 1964; Ibid., minute 8, by S.M.O. (T), 17 February 1964.
96. TNA BW 90/190 (Makerere University, Mulago Medical School and Hospital), Faculty of Medicine, Makerere College, 'Application to the Nuffield Foundation for the Services of a Visiting Consultant to Advise the College on Provision for Teaching and Research in Psychiatry and the Training of African Psychiatrists', April 1959, p. 1.
97. Ibid., p. 1.
98. Ibid., p. 2.
99. Ibid., p. 2.
100. A. W. Williams, 'The Next Generation', *East African Medical Journal* 34(10) (1957), pp. 521–528.
101. TNA BW 90/190, 'Application to the Nuffield Foundation', p. 2.
102. TNA BW 90/190, 'Application to the Nuffield Foundation', pp. 2–3.
103. BOD Mss.Afr.s.1872(153C) Part 1 (Papers of A. W. Williams), 'Reports, Memoranda, Offprints, etc.: Makerere Medical School, 1944–68', Item 7, D. L. Davies, 'Report on the Teaching of Psychiatry at Makerere College' (Unpublished report, Kampala, December 1959), p. 3.
104. Ibid.
105. Ibid., p. 13.
106. Ibid., pp. 5–6.
107. Ibid., p. 7.
108. Ibid., p. 13.
109. BOD Mss.Afr.s.1872(153C) Part 1, 'Reports, Memoranda, Offprints, etc.: Makerere Medical School, 1944–68', Item 8, 'Report of Principal's Psychiatry Committee', December 1960, p. 3.
110. Ibid., p. 12.
111. Iliffe, *East African Doctors*, p. 130.
112. BOD Mss.Afr.s.1872(153C) Part 1, 'Report of Principal's Psychiatry Committee', p. 16.
113. Uganda Protectorate, *Annual Report of the Medical Department for the Year Ended 31st December, 1958* (Entebbe, 1959), p. 79.
114. Personal communication with G. Allen German, 29 January 2012.
115. Personal communication with German; Personal communication with J. F. Wood, 7 October 2011.
116. BOD Mss.Afr.s.1872(153C) Part 1, 'Report of Principal's Psychiatry Committee', p. 2.
117. Ibid., pp. 7–8.

118. Personal communication with German.
119. Personal communication with Wilson Acuda, 21 October 2011; Personal communication with German; Personal communication with John Orley, 25 September 2011; and Personal communication with Wood.
120. See correspondence in UMOHA C90/ACR.
121. UMOHA ECC.29 (Consultants/Specialists—General), letter from I. S. Kadama, Chief Medical Officer, to Ian McAdam, Makerere Medical School, 6 September 1967; UMOHA ECC.29, minute from M/H to Chief Medical Officer, 8 January 1963; and TNA BW 90/190, letter from A. Williams to I. C. M. Maxwell, Inter-University Council, London, 29 April 1959.
122. 'Department of Psychiatry Annual Report, 1966–1967', *Makerere University College Reports, 1966–1967* (Kampala, copy in possession of author, 1967); 'Department of Psychiatry Annual Report, 1968–1969', *Makerere University College Reports, 1968–1969* (Kampala, copy in possession of author, 1969); Personal communication with German. In a study of psychiatric education in medical schools in the UK in 1967–1968, G. M. Carstairs et al. found that the mean number of hours devoted to psychiatric training was 185 hours. The range was 66 hours (Charing Cross) to 468 hours (Middlesex). G. M. Carstairs et al., 'Psychiatric Education: Survey of Undergraduate Psychiatric Teaching in the United Kingdom (1966–1967)', *British Journal of Psychiatry* 144 (1968), pp. 1411–1416.
123. D. L. Davies, 'Report on the Teaching of Psychiatry at Makerere University College Department of Psychiatry' (Unpublished report, copy in possession of author, 1969).
124. World Health Organization Archives (WHOA) M-PROJECTS UGANDA-38 (Assistance to the Department of Psychiatry, Makerere University College), 'Application to the World Health Organization for a Grant-in-Aid', 1966.
125. Personal communication with Wood.
126. J. F. Wood, 'Acute Brain Syndromes (or Organic Confusional States)' (Unpublished lecture, copy in possession of author, 1969).
127. Davies, 'Report on the Teaching of Psychiatry 1969'.
128. World Health Organization Library (WHOL) SEA/ME/Meet.Dir. Sch.P.H.4/23, 'Makerere University Medical School Country Report—Uganda, East Africa', p. 4.
129. 'Department of Psychiatry Annual Report, 1966–1967'; Personal communication with Orley.
130. Three months into his secondment, however, Aas suffered a major heart attack and died shortly afterwards. 'Department of Psychiatry Annual Report, 1968–1969'; Personal communication with German.

131. 'Department of Psychiatry Annual Report, 1968–1969'.
132. UMOHA C90/ACR, f. 81, note listing staff on duty and on leave at Butabika Hospital, 4 June 1964; 'Department of Psychiatry Annual Report, 1968–1969'; and Personal communication with German.
133. Personal communication with Acuda.
134. Personal communication with German.
135. UMOHA C90/ACR, f. 104, letter from J. Bulwanyi, Medical Superintendent, Butabika Hospital, to M. Kooyman, Medical Officer, and J. Muhangi, Medical Officer, 14 September 1966; Personal communication with German.
136. 'Department of Psychiatry Annual Report, 1966–1967'.
137. *Mental Health Services in the Developing World: Reports on Workshops on Mental Health, Edinburgh (1968) and Kampala (1969)*, Commonwealth Foundation Occasional Paper, IV (Hove, 1969), p. 51; Davies, 'Report on the Teaching of Psychiatry 1969'.
138. UMOHA C90/ACR, f. 134, letter from S. B. Bosa to Permanent Secretary for Establishments, Ministry of Public Service and Local Administration, 31 May 1972.
139. 'Department of Psychiatry Annual Report, 1966–1967'; 'Department of Psychiatry Annual Report, 1968–1969'.
140. Davies, 'Report on the Teaching of Psychiatry 1969'.
141. C. Sicherman, 'Building an African Department of History at Makerere, 1950–1972', *History in Africa* 30 (2003), p. 254.
142. W. D. Foster, 'Makerere Medical School: 50th Anniversary', *British Medical Journal* 3(5932) (1974), p. 678.
143. H. J. Simons, 'Mental Disease in Africans: Racial Determinism', *The British Journal of Psychiatry* 104(435) (1958), p. 387.
144. F. J. Bennett, 'Medical Manpower in East Africa: Prospects and Problems', *East African Medical Journal* 42(4) (1965), p. 154; Personal communication with Orley; and C. Sicherman, *Becoming an African University: Makerere, 1922–2000* (Trenton, 2005), Ch. 14.
145. Bennett, 'Medical Manpower in East Africa', p. 154.
146. UMOHA C90/ACR, f. 63, letter from Stephen Bosa to Dr. Davies, 22 June 1960.
147. Ibid.
148. Ibid.

CHAPTER 4

'Mass Hysteria' in the Wake of Decolonisation

In the early 1960s, medical officers and administrators in Uganda and Tanganyika (now Tanzania) began to receive reports of what was being described as 'mass madness' and 'mass hysteria' in the areas around Lake Victoria.[1] Starting with a case of 'laughing mania' at Bukoba, north–west Tanganyika, in 1962, further reports of 'running manias associated with violence' followed in 1963 in Kigezi, south–west Uganda, and Mbale, eastern Uganda. Faced with reports of up to 600 'victims' in each area, local medical officers were at a loss as to how to respond.[2] While they had well-established measures in place for investigating and preventing the spread of infectious diseases such as cerebrospinal meningitis, there were no guidelines dictating the proper procedure for a psychic epidemic. As an account in the *New York Times* noted: 'Near Bukoba an entire village of more than 200 persons fell ill in a matter of days .... To villagers with tears in the eyes from fits of hysteria, the disease is "endwara ya Kucheka"—the laughing trouble. To doctors, it is one of Africa's newest and most puzzling illnesses'.[3]

At the request of the Uganda and Tanganyika Governments, two different teams investigated the epidemics. The first, led by A. M. Rankin, Professor of Medicine at Makerere University College, and P. J. Philip, Medical Officer, described how a 'disease' of 'laughing, crying and restlessness' had started in 1962 at a mission-run girls' school twenty-five miles from Bukoba, Tanganyika.[4] In the subsequent months, the condition spread to other schools, affecting male and female pupils equally, but none of the European or African teachers. 'The onset is sudden', they noted, 'with attacks of laughing and crying lasting for a few minutes to a few hours, followed by a respite and then a recurrence. The attack is accompanied by restlessness and on occasions violence when restraint is attempted'.[5] They conducted a series of laboratory tests to rule out organic causes for the disorder, before reaching a tentative diagnosis of mass hysteria by process of elimination.[6] The second investigation was based at Mbale, eastern Uganda, and led by Benjamin H. Kagwa, who had returned to Uganda from the USA for two years in 1963. Kagwa conducted a series of neuropsychiatric tests, analysing his findings along-side historical examples of mass hysteria from sixteenth-century Europe. He showed little interest in local explanations for the madness, which linked it to the anger of ancestral spirits. Instead, Kagwa stressed that the epidemics, coming in the wake of independence from colonial rule, provided evidence that Africans were suffering from a 'mental conflict' brought on by education and 'westernisation'.[7] His research repre-sented the first major investigation into mental illness in East Africa by an African doctor.

The idea that Africans were prone to periodic outbursts of mass insta-bility had been present in medical and ethnographic literature since the mid-nineteenth century, and proliferated with the expansion of colonial rule.[8] Observers of the *amandiki* women in Zululand at the beginning of the twentieth century offered a number of different explanations for *indiki* possession, including witchcraft, healing cults and 'hysteri-cal mania'. In describing the behaviour of the *amandiki*, many colonial officials and missionaries also drew on the gendered language of hyste-ria that was prominent in Europe at the time.[9] In Nigeria in 1940, M. D. W. Jeffreys, a colonial administrative officer, included an outbreak of 'religious fervour' in the Calabar Province in his account of 'psychical phenomena' in Africans. 'Victims', he noted, 'declared themselves pos-sessed of the spirit and giving way to paroxysms of dancing finally collapsed in insensibility which usually ended in a return to sanity. Large masses moved about the country singing religious hymns'.[10] In Kenya, too, ethnologists described how 'psychical disturbances of a religious character pass like epidemics over the Kamba country'. These distur-bances, known locally as *kijesu*, were categorised variously as 'infectious hysteria' and 'epidemic mania', and were given a distinctly political tone—at Ulu, according to Gerhard Lindblom, people went into convulsions at the mere sight of a European.[11] Such accounts formed part of a broader attempt to describe and define what constituted 'normal' and 'abnormal' behaviour in the African. Infusing their work with notions of European racial and cultural superiority, authors dismissed indigenous cultural practices and beliefs as evidence of psychopathology. As Megan Vaughan has argued, the distinction between witchcraft and madness was frequently blurred: 'It was 'normal' (if punishable) for an African to believe in witchcraft—it was not 'normal', however, to suffer from paranoid delusions'.[12] Yet such was the power of these beliefs, it was said, that Africans could will themselves to die.[13]

The epidemic nature of so-called psychic disturbances was particularly worrying for medical practitioners and colonial administrators: if unchecked, mass instability had the potential to spread and destabilise whole regions.[14] These fears were reinforced from the 1920s and 1930s, when psychologists and anthropologists within the East African School of Psychiatry and Psychology started to discuss how education and urbanisation could 'detribalise' the African and trigger a particularly 'European' type of insanity, characterised by delusions of power and control.[15] Such ideas were certainly present in reports on 'outbreaks' of mass fervour and spirit cults in Uganda, where they operated as useful explanatory tools. One of the most threatening movements for administrators in early colonial Uganda was that of the fertility goddess *Nyabingi* in Kigezi District, characterised by contemporary observers as an anti-colonial 'society' or 'cult', and refigured more recently as a set of logics and practices associated with attempts to gain redress for misfortune.[16] In one of the most notorious incidents linked to *Nyabingi*, a horde of Kiga men and women stormed the local government station at Nyakishenyi, killing sixty-three government employees and family members working under the supervision of a colonial agent from Buganda. Responding to the attack in a report in 1917, the District Commissioner (DC) of Kigezi District, J. M. M. McDougall, dismissed the suggestion that the rebellion indicated anti-Ganda or even anti-colonial sentiment.[17] Instead, witchcraft was to blame: 'As might be expected among unsophisticated savages the powers of superstition are enormous. This explains the influence of the local witchdoctors, who initially combine their claims to supernatural powers with promises of liberation of the natives from European rule and restoration to their former condition'.[18]

Two years later, a new DC, Captain J. E. T. Philipps, updated this theory, drawing on ideas about hypnotism and unconscious suggestion. For Philipps, *Nyabingi* practices were spreading '[by] means of an unusually developed form of Witchcraft, in which hypnotic suggestion plays a leading part, the country within the sphere of its operations is completely terrorised'.[19]

Such accounts of mass instability during colonial rule tell us more about the anxieties and vulnerability of the colonial project than they do about the behaviours and actions of those involved. They overlook personal testimonies, and the ways such behaviours might also be read as forms of protest, as expressions of wider social and political anxieties, or as ways of coping with distress within evolving frameworks of healing. Whether such behaviours are labelled 'mass hysteria' or not, they are always subject to multiple, shifting opinions and explanations, of which (Western) medical diagnosis is only one part. This is no less the case for the epidemics of 'mass hysteria' that emerged in the early 1960s, for which the medical reports obscure the wider socio-economic and political disruption of decolonisation. Rankin, Philip, and Kagwa, among others, could have found plenty of tensions and potential causes of conflict, had they looked for them. Indeed, the broader emotional landscape of Uganda in the run-up to Independence in 1962 was one of 'widespread passionate politics', to borrow a phrase from Carol Summers.[20] Nationalist and monarchical politics became more vocal across Uganda through the 1950s, with multiple competing local interests undermining hopes of a 'unified' nation state, and prompting uncertainty about the future. One of the most prominent political confrontations resulted from the colonial government's exiling of Buganda's *Kabaka* (King) Mutesa II to London in November 1953, following increasingly tense discussions about plans for an East African federation. The 'Kabaka crisis' of 1953–1955 saw public demonstrations of grief and loyalty, with Ganda women weeping openly in the streets.[21] What was more worrying for the colonial government, however, was what they interpreted as a 'resurgence' of spirit possession practices, particularly in the already emotionally charged context of the Kabaka crisis.[22] The *lubaale* (hero-god) prophet Kigaanira Ssewannyana, channelling the principal *lubaale* of warfare, *Kibuuka*, openly contested colonial authority by urging the Ganda to withhold taxes until the return of the exiled Kabaka, to stop attending church and mosque services, and by handing out his own medicines.[23] Kigaanira was eventually arrested amidst violence between his supporters and the police, culminating in the death of the Head Constable of the Buganda Native Police.

Psychiatry occupied a marginal space in these upheavals of decolonisation. Aside from the extension of responsibility to Ugandan psychiatrists, as examined in the previous chapter, psychiatry saw little change—the number of patients admitted to Mulago and Butabika Mental Hospitals continued to rise, and there was no overhaul of diagnostic or therapeutic practices. When Kigaanira was charged with murder following his arrest, his defence of insanity was rejected by the High Court of Uganda and the medical practitioners who examined him.[24] As political tensions continued into the 1960s, moreover, including ongoing conflict between the Uganda Government and the Buganda Kingdom, and the collapse of constitutional governance, psychiatry remained insular.[25] This was no less the case in eastern Uganda, where administrative restructuring and controversies surrounding circumcision saw the Gisu of eastern Uganda develop a reputation for extreme violence.

This chapter uses the 'mass madness' that swept across the Mbale region of eastern Uganda in the early 1960s as a lens through which to explore the place of psychiatry in the context of political instability. In situating the epidemic in its wider social and political context, I aim not only to explore how broader anxieties may have found expression in spirit possession, but also to highlight the difficulties facing the first generation of Ugandan psychiatrists as they took over responsibility for psychiatry. Responses to the epidemic remind us that the practice of psychiatry was not necessarily transformed with the emergence of African psychiatrists, even if contemporaries had credited them with having natural cultural 'insight' into 'the African mind'. Psychiatrists like Kagwa found it just as difficult as their expatriate colleagues to bridge what Frederick Cooper and Ann Laura Stoler have called 'the stretch between the public institutions of the colonial state and the intimate reaches of people's lives'.[26] Not only did their education, class and language skills set them apart from their patients, but there remained fundamental differences between their understandings of mental illness and the types of treatment deemed to be effective.

ANXIETIES IN THE WAKE OF DECOLONISATION

In the years following Independence in 1962, administrative structures at the local level were dismantled as Prime Minister Milton Obote and the Uganda People's Congress (UPC) attempted to assert their control over the districts.[27] The reorganisation of boundaries came as no surprise to officials in eastern Uganda, where territorial claims over Mbale Town had resulted in growing tensions through the 1950s. In 1954, Mbale had been designated as the administrative centre of two districts, Bugisu and Bukedi, with both the Gisu and Gwere (the main ethnic groups in these two districts, respectively) keen to secure ownership of the town. In these disputes, as Pamela Khanakwa has shown, *imbalu* (circumcision) practices, and associated discourses of manhood and the traditionally circumcised male body, were invoked by Gisu administrators and nationalists as a way of undermining the territorial claims of the Gwere, who were uncircumcised. This conflict over Mbale led to riots in 1954 and 1956, during which a number of Gwere and uncircumcised Gisu men were forcibly circumcised.[28] In the following years, the region saw a spate of forced circumcisions, as well as increasing tension, as Uganda headed towards independence with the Mbale question still unresolved. In June 1962, when the Boundary Commission was considering the Bugisu/Bugwere boundary dispute, 300–400 Gisu, including large numbers of *imbalu* dancers, gathered in protest, prompting the police to respond with tear gas and gunfire.[29] Anxieties about *imbalu* were felt throughout the region. In 1964, Israel K., an elderly man visiting the Bubule Health Centre with a scrotal hernia, appealed for help from the District Medical Officer for protection from neighbours who he feared were planning to forcibly circumcise him.[30]

Against this backdrop of political instability, the Mbale region—already densely populated—saw increasing pressure on land, as well as fluctuating coffee prices, contributing to a perception that theft, bhang growing, drinking, witchcraft, and violence were getting out of control.[31] Highlighting the complex relationship between political authority and generational tensions, the Intelligence Committee noted in 1964 that 'the traditional customs and superstitions which tamed the man to abide by certain rules of laws have disappeared. Religio[n]s which have been brought in by foreign powers are heavily under criticism and losing ground. Many fathers have lost the old control that they used to have over their children. Drunkenness has increased with little criticism from parents'.[32] Such was the extent of fear over these issues that from the mid-1960s two types of neighbourhood organisations—vigilante groups and drinking companies—were formed across the area in order to curb social activities that were deemed to be dangerous.[33] The local administration, too, started to meet regularly to question how they could respond to the rising homicide rate and general unrest in the area. One proposed approach was to increase agricultural activity in the area. Yet, as a frustrated District Agricultural Officer, F. X. Lubega, complained in June 1965, this approach was futile 'because it is not basically an agricultural problem'.[34]

If tensions in eastern Uganda prompted mass action or healing in the form of a protest cult, it was not recognised as such by anthropologists, psychiatrists or those affected. Nevertheless, Gisu elders living in the area surrounding Mbale recalled that there was a time around *kukwihula* (Independence) when madness was common, when 'so many people were attacked around the villages', and it was 'catching many people in one go'.[35] The madness (*tsitsoli*) was said to have come suddenly during the years immediately preceding and following Independence, lasted a few months, and never recurred. It was as if mass madness, as a number of elders described it, was a 'disease of that time' (*lufu lwembuka yo*), just as HIV/AIDS is regarded as a 'disease of today'.[36] This way of remembering both indicates the extent to which it had affected families and communities, and points to the ways Gisu elders periodise time by major events and disturbances. Gisu circumcision names (*kamengilo*), for example, were usually associated with social, economic and political events.[37] In reflection of the spate of forced circumcisions, the 1966 circumcision name was *muwambe*, meaning 'capture, catch or hold him'.[38]

'It came by wind [*imbewo*]', as a Gisu elder described it.[39] Just as the *basambwa* (ancestral spirits) were 'like the wind', so the madness was said to have come and spread in this way.[40] In describing the madness, a number of explanations were put forward, including a curse from the ancestors and witchcraft (*liloko* and *bulosi*).[41] 'It was a result of misfortunes [*bisilani*], because it came as wind and people contracted it', posited one Gisu elder.[42] 'In our area', another stressed, 'people said it was a curse [*shitsubo*]'.[43] Speaking about his own madness during the epidemic, moreover, one man remained uncertain about why he was affected: 'I don't know, maybe it came by spirits [*were*]. But what I know, is that it affected many people'.[44] While it was more common among the youth, it did not discriminate by gender, education or age.[45] This, according to a number of elders, was due to the will of *were*, the creator spirit.[46] No contradiction was seen in the diversity of explanations—ideas about agency behind the madness reflected the more general belief that while *were* (the creator spirit) was in charge of fate, agency could be ascribed to sorcery, the anger of the ancestors, or other spirits.[47] As one elder commented, 'Everybody had his or her own theory, because some said it came from the ancestors and others, that it was a curse from God'.[48]

In line with the broader unrest in the region, as well as ethnographic accounts of madness among the Gisu, violence and aggression were cited as key features of the behaviour of those affected.[49] 'He was very much aggressive and sometimes silent', one informant spoke of a man in a neighbouring village. Such was his confusion in his final days, she added, that he wandered into the path of a vehicle and was killed.[50] Others might 'cry too much, become aggressive, become quiet, or laugh too much'.[51] Or they might 'become very violent and would keep away from noise or cry uncontrollably'.[52] Those who went mad themselves, however, offered different views. 'At times I would feel like I was losing my senses', one Gisu elder recalled, 'and sometimes could not trace my home'.[53] Another reported how it gave her headaches and left her 'quiet' and 'docile'.[54] What was clear was that the scale of the madness caused considerably anxiety, with reports of rumours about its spread moving between villages, particularly during periods of *imbalu*.[55] On hearing a rumour, one elder explained, 'Some people became scared and isolated themselves'.[56] While another, speaking of her own disturbance, recalled feeling isolated, adding that 'People became scared that if they came near they would be affected'.[57]

In a context in which there was some uncertainty over the cause and spread of the madness, rumours flourished, pointing to anxieties that transcended local politics. One theory was that the scale of the madness was due to 'sophisticated bombs', something that may have reflected heavy news coverage on nuclear testing (including that within Africa) at the time.[58] Another, perhaps related idea, was that it had come from 'outside', as an unknown force from Europe.[59] Fears about nuclear testing, and its effects, certainly linked the epidemic to that in Tanganyika, where Rankin and Philip reported a 'belief that the atmosphere has been poisoned as a result of the atom bomb explosions'.[60] Yet it also highlighted uncertainties about the intentions and actions of foreigners. One Gisu elder recalled two Europeans coming to investigate the local water supply at the same time as people in his and nearby villages were running mad. These Europeans, he believed, were only interested in the water because the madness had 'started from abroad....In countries like Germany'.[61] This explanation might be best attributed to anxieties about the nature of medical research and colonial rule.[62] But it might also be taken as an indication of the cultural and political gulf between the Gisu, the local authorities, and foreign researchers. What for the two Europeans was a routine and unobtrusive water test, became for this man something altogether more disturbing. Indeed, because the Europeans 'knew about the disease', they could avoid being infected, having 'covered themselves with protective masks'.[63]

The extent to which Gisu elders recalled uncertainty and suspicion, both towards the behaviours they witnessed and the people who came to investigate, remind us that historians should not focus solely on diagnosis. Yet proving, 'without doubt', the diagnosis of mass hysteria was a foremost concern for Kagwa when he arrived to investigate the epidemic in 1964.[64] In doing so, Kagwa would show little interest in local explanations for the madness or the wider social and political context in which it emerged and took hold.

The 'Problem' of Mass Hysteria

Kagwa returned to Uganda in August 1963 on the invitation of the newly independent Ministry of Health. It was his first visit home after thirty-five years overseas, and driven, according to his wife, Winifred Kagwa, by a 'moral responsibility' to 'contribute to the development of his homeland'.[65] Indeed, it was the political upheavals of decolonisation, and their effects on mental health, that had concerned Kagwa. In the context of conflict in Congo and the 'new winds of change in Africa', he wrote in his memoir, 'it would be a shame if I shunned the responsibility of offering my services where they are acutely needed'.[66] In Uganda, he noted, 'one sees a mixture of poverty and prosperity, cleanliness, and boiling political as well as intellectual activities'.[67] And the political situation was changing quickly: 'Since I have been here many things have happened: the king of Buganda has become the *President* of *Uganda*. Kenya has become independent. A group of Europeans organized by some Kenya-born whites to mock the Kenya *Uhuru* on Ugandan soil were summarily deported, and the concept of the Rhodesian federation is dead, bringing about the resurrection of Nyasaland (Malawi) and Northern Rhodesia (Zambia) as living entities preparing for whooping *Uhurus*'.[68]

Between 1963 and 1965, Kagwa was on 'safari', as he termed it, as a consultant psychiatrist for the Uganda Government. Joining Stephen B. Bosa and T. W. Murray as Uganda's only psychiatrists before 1966, Kagwa divided his time between Mulago and Butabika Hospitals, and took on inspection visits to hospitals across the country. Yet while Bosa was unable to take any leave due to pressures on his workload, Kagwa's memoir speaks (in the manner of other doctor memoirs of Africa), of visits with his wife to the source of the Nile, Murchison Falls National Park, Nairobi, Mombasa, Zanzibar and Ngorongoro Crater, where they encountered a rhino 'on the loose' in their camp.[69] Refuting any notions of savagery, and continuing an ongoing preoccupation in his memoir with beautiful women, he stressed how 'it is markedly difficult in Kampala to find a sloppily dressed woman...always gorgeously dressed and meticulously neat'.[70] 'Maybe I shouldn't say this', he added, 'but one day I made a remark about my impression of the neatness of the Kampala African woman to a clinician in the large city hospital who has been examining them for years. His remark was, "Even their underwear is clean"'.[71]

Despite his expressed interest in the relationship between decolonisation and mental health, Kagwa's reflections on his clinical experiences received significantly less attention in his memoir than comments about scenery, socialising and African women. Nevertheless, he noted his surprise at how similar the symptomatology of psychotics and psycho-neurotics was to that encountered in the USA. It was only in the content of the delusions that differences, or 'local cultural shades', could be found. While in the USA 'paranoids...may express their ideas of reference by saying that the neighbors are sending some radio waves or electricity through their bodies, trying to kill them', in Uganda, 'paranoids...substitute magic for radio waves'.[72] Such comments echoed the preoccupations of colonial psychiatrists with understanding differences between 'African' and 'European' delusions, but were much more in line with the emergent stream within transcultural psychiatry that saw mental illness as both universal and shaped by culture. The idea that there might be syndromes bound by culture was also an area of fascination. He wrote how a series of neuropsychiatric cases, 'which do not fit in any pathological or clinical entities I have known in the USA', presented themselves as 'peculiar "tough nuts", but they are evocative and stimulating to study'.[73]

Kagwa's interest in the epidemics of 'mass hysteria' sweeping across eastern Africa marked the conflation of his interest in culture-bound syndromes and the political upheavals of decolonisation, and with permission from the Uganda Government, he travelled to Mbale to investigate. In describing the epidemic of 'running mania', Kagwa divided the madness into three stages. The first came on suddenly and lasted three to four days. It was characterised by 'marked agitation, talkativeness, violence, attempted assaults and petty robbery, with anorexia and a craving to smoke'.[74] The second was marked by sporadic relapses of hyperactivity, lasting one to two weeks. And the third was characterised by 'improvement in mood, affability and a willingness to be interviewed'.[75] According to his research, all of the original cases were Gisu men and women, either illiterate or near-illiterate, and in no position of authority.[76]

In discussing possible causes for the outbreak, Kagwa noted that those affected believed very strongly that the madness was caused by ancestral spirits. 'All this was said to be done', Kagwa asserted, 'in response to the orders of the spirits of dead family elders. This phase had a quality of a quasi-manic reaction with obvious transparent delusions and hallucinations. Those affected stated that they could see the faces and hear the voices of their dead elders'.[77] Surprisingly, Kagwa did not pursue this line of inquiry, or consider the broader context of political instability in the Mbale region, despite expressing sympathy for prominent psychoanalysts such as Sigmund Freud, who argued that an individual or group's ideas, fears and anxieties could produce hysteria.[78] Instead, he initiated a series of invasive physical and neuropsychiatric tests that included lumbar punctures, hypnosis, drug abreaction and the pushing of pins an inch deep into the flesh in order to show total anaesthesia.[79] Ignoring the possibility that his actions might in themselves cause distress, Kagwa asserted that his tests and interviews showed 'several objective classical hysterical findings'. These included 'sudden onset of the attacks, sudden clearance of symptoms', and total numbness. For Kagwa, 'all clinical studies proved, without doubt, the diagnosis of conversion hysteria'.[80]

In making this statement, Kagwa was using his examination of individuals to diagnose the collective. This he justified by noting that 'one striking feature' of the three epidemics across East Africa was 'the stereotypy of symptoms in each particular ethnological group. The "attacks" and spread of similar symptoms ran along tribal lines. Even in instances where it spread over geographical borders the epidemics affected only members of the same tribe and culture'.[81] The statements mirrored those made by Rankin and Philip in their investigation of the epidemic in Tanganyika, which had stressed that mental illness was 'influenced by the culture of the particular community'.[82] Yet while Rankin and Philip were reluctant to draw further conclusions before a study of the cultural context in Bukoba had been undertaken, Kagwa was more confident of his understanding of mental illness across East Africa. As a psychiatrist—and an African one at that—he not only confirmed that these epidemics were linked, but that they had implications for political, social and economic stability in the region—epidemics of mass hysteria were a new East African 'problem'. In his analysis, Kagwa would fall back on many of the assumptions of the East African School of Psychiatry and Psychology, and would conflate ethnicity and culture with race.

Kagwa drew heavily on J. C. Carothers' notion that the introduction of Western culture into Africa was upsetting an 'equilibrium', and that Africans were ill-equipped, both culturally and environmentally, to cope with these changes.[83] Echoing Carothers, Kagwa noted that:

> Consciously or unconsciously, at this period of their development, the majority of Africans have conflicts of great psychological dimensions, though they may differ in character. For example, among the educated the conflict may be verbalized in terms of political, economic or educational unrest and action, while among the illiterate and near-illiterate confusion of ideas and emotions, as well as substitution of mysticism for logic, is the rule....the latter group, which is of course in the majority, has been thrust into sudden religious and political changes without preparation.[84]

Kagwa's use of Carothers is not entirely surprising given the continued interest of psychiatrists and psychologists in the idea of the African in transition. While statements about the dangers of 'development' and other assumptions of ethnopsychiatry were increasingly being contested, not least by African psychiatrists such as T. A. Lambo, ethnopsychiatry nevertheless represented the only substantial body of literature on African psychopathology.[85] Moreover, the World Health Organization (WHO), which had commissioned Carothers' *The African Mind in Health and Disease*, stood publicly by the text as late as 1962 as a 'good example' of an investigation 'of the peculiar qualities of mental organization in individual cultural groups'.[86]

Despite his reliance on ideas about 'psychic trauma', 'culture contact', and 'detribalisation', Kagwa certainly believed that his investigation was less racially motivated than that which had come before under colonial rule. Significantly, Kagwa was keen to stress that his analysis did not mean that mass hysteria was a cultural or racial peculiarity affecting Africans alone. Discussing the historical background of mass hysteria, Kagwa noted that 'Hysteria, as a human behavioural phenomenon, can be traced as far back as the beginning of man's rational psycho-social development'; it was functional, providing an 'outlet for dammed-up instinctive demands'.[87] In doing so, Kagwa stressed the universal applicability of Western psychiatry alongside the existence of a linear scale of development on which African 'civilisation' was passing through one stage. There was 'much historical evidence', Kagwa added, 'to prove that emotional upheavals associated with hysteria occur whenever a people's cultural roots and beliefs become suddenly shattered'.[88] These precedents included demon possession in the Bible, the hysterical deliria of saints, and epidemics of dancing mania in Metz, Cologne and Aix-la-Chapelle in the fourteenth and fifteenth centuries.[89]

By including these examples Kagwa was following a trend in medicine of analysing historical accounts of disease, as if it might aid understanding of why and when epidemics of hysteria occur.[90] In ways reminiscent of older theories of recapitulation, this body of literature linked the 'primitive' mentalities of peasants from medieval Europe with twentieth-century schoolchildren, members of religious cults and black Americans, among others. The problem with this approach was the way it assumed that mass hysteria had always existed in a universal and recognisable form, and that retrospective diagnoses could shed light on present understandings.[91] Indeed, for Kagwa, as it had been for Rankin and Philip, mass hysteria was an objective reality; it could spread from person to person just as other types of epidemic disease were 'caused by the spread of viruses, bacteria or parasites'.[92]

Despite Kagwa's attempts to distance himself from ideas about racial difference, he could not escape the assumption that African societies were undergoing a period of psychological transition. He saw no contradiction between his finding that the epidemics ran along ethnic lines and his belief in the existence of a homogenous African culture that was, at this particular time, susceptible to mass instability. This 'African culture' was the only useful unit of analysis, just as it had been for Carothers—there was little room for socio-economic change, cultural diversity or individuality. It was Kagwa's attempt to understand the epidemics through this particular theoretical lens that accounts for the conceptual gap between him and his Gisu patients.

MULTIPLE RESPONSES TO 'MASS MADNESS'

These different ways of 'seeing' and understanding psychological distress were not resolved with the coming of Independence or with the emergence of African psychiatrists. Kagwa may have been an African by birth, but he was from central rather than eastern Uganda, and his years in the USA had further distanced him from the people he was trying to help. As Kagwa noted later, he had returned to Uganda with a set of assumptions about the African mind that were rooted in Western psychiatric theory, rather than any special insight derived from being Ugandan.[93] His analysis of the epidemic as a wider cultural and developmental issue stands starkly against the social, political and economic tensions that existed in the area, as well as the explanations of the Gisu. In spite of this, or perhaps because of it, there remained a large question mark over how the 'problem' of mass hysteria should be handled.

If Kagwa believed in the universal applicability of psychiatry for understanding mental illness, he was nevertheless aware of the limits of his power. A Psychiatric Unit to serve the Eastern Region had opened at Mbale Hospital in 1963–1964, staffed by a small group of psychiatric nurses, but only four beds were available during the period under question.[94] Kagwa, moreover, was only able to apply his neuropsychiatric 'test' to those in the recovery stage of the epidemic, and does not appear to have been allowed to offer his own treatments. Just because Kagwa was Ugandan, it did not mean that families and communities were any more likely to turn to him for help. Such were the limits of Kagwa's role in Mbale that he was left to describe how it was Gisu elders 'who perform the healing ritual'.[95] These elders, Kagwa continued:

> start at sunrise by visiting the burial grounds of the clan and by weeding the tombs, near which they build small huts. White chickens are slaughtered and their blood used to anoint the tombs. Pieces of chicken, baked plantains and calabashes of wine are then placed in the huts. These are gifts to the spirits of dead clan elders. Finally, one elder sips the wine and spits it on the feet of the "possessed", who then becomes instantaneously and dramatically healed. Interestingly enough, the word for this ritual is equivalent to the English word "exorcism".[96]

Kagwa's account fit with that described by anthropologist Jean La Fontaine on the sacrificing of white animals to 'good' spirits and to the ancestors.[97] By focusing on the dramatic, however, such accounts ignored the importance of other forms of healing, including herbs, protective charms and even Western medicine.

Like other ethnic groups in Uganda, the Gisu distinguished between the symptomatic and etiological treatment of illness, focusing first on relieving symptoms before looking for a deeper cause.[98] Herbal medicine was easily available and regarded as the first line of treatment in cases of sickness.[99] One of those affected by the madness described visiting a healer who specialised in herbs. This healer, he noted, was relied upon because of their proximity and because through herbal medicine, 'they had seen other victims heal'. While it took some time before he recovered, he credited his own health to that of the herbalist, and the support of his family.[100] Those seeking relief could also turn to other forms of medicine, including protective charms (*tsisale*) placed under the skin, and ritual specialists who had the ability to remove bad omens and curses.[101] The methods and meetings of these specialists were usually highly secretive, but could include sacrifices to appease the spirits or to drive out misfortune.[102] Western medicine was also an option for those seeking relief and, despite the long distances that needed to be travelled, a number of people visited hospitals and clinics at Mbale and Bududu.[103] One woman recalled how they would only initiate treatment when people became aggressive, and then a person would either be tied up, taken to hospital, a traditional healer, or left to die. One of her neighbours, she added, was first taken to the government hospital at Mbale, in part because it was not far from their home, but also because that was what their village chief encouraged them to do. This particular person recovered in the hospital, and as a result, others from her village were also taken there for treatment.[104]

Distance was a key factor in the decision-making process for those affected by the epidemic. More often than not, distances were perceived to be too great,[105] particularly for those who were not convinced of the ability of Western medicine to deal with illnesses associated with ancestral spirits.[106] A few also regarded hospitals as places of danger, in the way Luise White has highlighted more generally for East and Central Africa.[107] 'Some people had a false belief', one Gisu elder recalled, 'that in hospitals medicines were made out of dead people'.[108] Such a comment reveals concern over the power of European therapies, and the control that was felt over bodies and minds.

As elsewhere in Africa, it was families and the larger kinship group who played a central role in making decisions about care and treatment, displaying a pragmatism that allowed for alternative treatment options to be explored.[109] As John Orley noted on his experience of illness and disease in central Uganda, 'Africans, being pragmatists, looked for a system that worked, and if one traditional remedy failed then another could be tried and so on until eventually Western medical treatment could also be given its chance'.[110] Among the Gisu, such was the extent of this pragmatism that different methods of treatment were used simultaneously. One woman, for example, described how her brother was among those who went mad, becoming extremely aggressive and feeling cold to the touch. As a family they had first taken him to Mbale Hospital, but then decided that in addition to Western medicine, they would also consult two different traditional healers. When questioned as to why they tried three kinds of treatment 'at a go', she laughed, before responding: 'We wanted him to get cured'.[111] This was not a question of selecting traditional or Western medicine, but rather a process of searching for relief.

CONCLUSION

The epidemics of the early 1960s indicate the limits, rather than the strengths of psychiatry during the upheavals of decolonisation. In the context of anxieties over nationalist politics, territorial claims and increasing violence, psychiatric practices ignored the social, focusing instead on individual, largely physical examinations of patients. Kagwa not only obscured the broader context of political instability, but also appeared unaware of the widespread uncertainty and suspicion about the epidemic, both in terms of the behaviours communities had to deal with, and the strangers who came to investigate. Rather than seeing decolonisation through the lens of the social, he presented Gisu explanations for distress as signs of psychopathology. Like psychiatrists and psychologists before him, moreover, he believed it was possible to generalise about mental illness in Africa, as well as to identify broad cultural traits and 'experiences'. While Kagwa certainly believed that he was contributing to a deracialisation of psychiatric theory, he was not able to free himself fully from the assumptions that had pervaded his discipline under colonial rule. This rendered psychiatry irrelevant. When the Gisu looked for options for relief, they turned to their own methods of healing—methods that did not include psychiatry. Kagwa, himself an outsider, was unable to intervene, his role reduced from psychiatric expert to that of observer.

While Kagwa's reliance on psychiatrists like Carothers placed him firmly within a much longer tradition of psychiatry in East Africa, it would be unfair to present Kagwa as an anomaly among the new generation of African psychiatrists emerging elsewhere in Africa. Intellectually, Kagwa navigated an uneasy line, being on the one hand a neuropsychiatrist with training in psychoanalysis, and on the other a visitor to a continent where many of the assumptions of ethnopsychiatry had yet to be fully unpicked by psychiatrists. Even the most critical of the early African psychiatrists, Lambo, found it difficult to navigate a path through the categories and terminologies employed by ethnopsychiatrists.[112] Over the next decade, the epidemics of mass hysteria also became a focus for transcultural psychiatrists working both within and outside of Africa. Moving beyond Kagwa's interest in the peculiarities of the African psyche, these discussions not only questioned why such epidemics occurred, but what they revealed about treatment choices in different cultural settings. At a Ciba Foundation Symposium on Transcultural Psychiatry, held in London in 1965, the events in East Africa were compared with epidemics of mass hysteria among islanders from Tristan da Cunha, *ufufenyane* among the Zulu in South Africa and Beatlemania.[113] Lambo, who claimed to have worked with Kagwa on his investigation, stressed that the finding that most people took their relatives to traditional healers was significant. Highlighting the 'differences between an African physician...with a completely Western medical education and the local therapists', Lambo observed how '[a] rural African coming from his village to consult me may say to himself: "Well, this man won't really have any sympathy with me, I will not come next time. I'm wasting my time with him"'.[114]

By the mid-1960s, the initial optimism that had accompanied calls for the training of Africans as psychiatrists had faded away. The question of how psychiatrists in Africa—both African and expatriate—could bridge the gap between Western psychiatry and African patients would come to dominate the agendas of pan-African conferences and workshops over the next twenty years. This would in turn raise further questions about the training of other health and medical workers in mental health care, the place of traditional healers in psychiatry, and whether psychiatrists could—and indeed should—take on social advisory roles in newly independent countries. The problem of the distance between psychiatrists and patients was, of course, not limited to the African context. In the UK, where psychiatrists were drawn almost exclusively from the upper echelons of society, the 1960s saw a proliferation of studies highlighting the difficulties of communication across class, education and linguistic divides.[115] Given the formative nature of the discipline of psychiatry in Africa, however, the problems experienced by psychiatrists in demonstrating the relevance of psychiatry took on particular significance during the late 1960s and early 1970s. It was through discussions among those working in the continent, as much as in new research conducted by psychiatrists, that the future of mental health services in developing countries started to be debated and reformed.

NOTES

1. An earlier version of this chapter was published as Y. Pringle, 'Investigating "Mass Hysteria" in Early Postcolonial Uganda: Benjamin H. Kagwa, East African Psychiatry, and the Gisu', *Journal of the History of Medicine and Allied Sciences* 70(1) (2015), pp. 105–136. I thank Oxford University Press for permission to reproduce some of this material here.

2. Kabale District Archives (KDA), Minutes of the Kigezi District Team, August 1963–July 1964; 'Mystery of the Laughing and Crying Disease', *Uganda Argus*, 15 August 1963, p. 3; G. J. Ebrahim, 'Mass Hysteria in School Children: Notes on Three Outbreaks in East Africa', *Afya* 3(10) (1969), pp. 7–9; B. H. Kagwa, 'The Problem of Mass Hysteria in East Africa', *East African Medical Journal* 41 (1964), pp. 560–566; and A. M. Rankin and P. J. Philip, 'An Epidemic of Laughing in the Bukoba District of Tanganyika', *The Central African Journal of Medicine* 9(5) (1963), pp. 167–170.

3. R. Conley, 'Laughing Malady Puzzle in Africa', *New York Times*, 8 August 1963, p. 29.

4. Rankin and Philip, 'An Epidemic of Laughing', p. 168.

5. Ibid., p. 167.

6. Ibid., pp. 167–170.

7. KDA, Minutes of the Kigezi District Team, August 1963–July 1964; 'Mystery of the Laughing and Crying Disease', p. 3; Conley, 'Laughing

Malady Puzzle'; Ebrahim, 'Mass Hysteria in School Children'; Kagwa, 'The Problem of Mass Hysteria'; and Rankin and Philip, 'An Epidemic of Laughing'.

8. One of the earliest is: A. Davidson, 'Choreomania: An Historical Sketch, with Some Account of an Epidemic Observed in Madagascar', *Edinburgh Medical Journal* XIII (1867), pp. 131–132.

9. J. Parle, *States of Mind: Searching for Mental Health in Natal and Zululand, 1868–1918* (Scottsville, 2007).

10. M. D. W. Jeffreys, 'Psychical Phenomena Among Negroes', *Journal of the Royal African Society* (1940), p. 355.

11. G. Lindblom, *The Akamba in British East Africa: An Ethnological Monograph* (Uppsala, 1920), p. 239. For a fuller treatment of *kijesu* see S. Mahone, 'The Psychology of Rebellion: Colonial Medical Responses to Dissent in British East Africa', *Journal of African History* 47(2) (2006), pp. 243–244.

12. M. Vaughan, *Curing Their Ills: Colonial Power and African Illness* (Cambridge, 1991), p. 106. See also Parle, *States of Mind*, Ch. 3.

13. See, for example, M. Wrong, 'Mass Education in Africa', *African Affairs* (1944), p. 109.

14. Mahone, 'The Psychology of Rebellion'.

15. J. C. Carothers, 'A Study of Mental Derangement in Africans, and an Attempt to Explain Its Peculiarities, More Especially in Relation to the African Attitude to Life', *East African Medical Journal* 25(5) (1948), pp. 142–166, 197–219; Vaughan, *Curing Their Ills*, Ch. 5.

16. R. Vokes, *Ghosts of Kanungu: Fertility, Secrecy & Exchange in the Great Lakes of East Africa* (Kampala, 2009), Ch. 2.

17. F. S. Brazier, 'The Incident at Nyakishenyi, 1917', *Uganda Journal* 32(1) (1968), pp. 17–27; Vokes, *Ghosts of Kanungu*, pp. 35–36.

18. E. Hopkins, 'The Nyabingi Cult of Southwestern Uganda', in R. I. Rotberg and A. A. Mazrui, eds., *Protest and Power in Black Africa* (New York, 1970), p. 291.

19. As cited in H. B. Hansen, 'The Colonial Control of Spirit Cults in Uganda', in D. M. Anderson and D. H. Johnson, eds., *Revealing Prophets: Prophecy in Eastern African History* (London, 1995), p. 154. On *Nyabingi* see especially S. Feierman, 'Colonizers, Scholars, and the Creation of Invisible Histories', in V. E. Bonnell and L. Hunt, eds., *Beyond the Cultural Turn: New Directions in the Study of Society and Culture* (Berkeley and Los Angeles, 1999); and Vokes, *Ghosts of Kanungu*.

20. C. Summers, 'All the Kabaka's Wives: Marital Claims in Buganda's 1953–5 Kabaka Crisis', *The Journal of African History* 58(1) (2017), p. 108.

21. Summers, 'All the Kabaka's Wives'. See also, P. Kavuma, *Crisis in Buganda, 1953–55: The Story of the Exile and Return of the Kabaka, Mutesa II* (London, 1979).

22. The National Archives, Kew, United Kingdom (TNA) CO 822/1191 (Neo-Paganism in Uganda), Special Branch Report: 'The Reversion from Christianity in Uganda', December 1955.

23. See reports in TNA CO 822/812 (Disturbances Caused by the Activities of a Young Muganda "Mathias", in Uganda). See also, J. L. Earle, 'Political Theologies in Late Colonial Buganda' (PhD thesis, University of Cambridge, 2012), pp. 256–263; N. Kodesh, *Beyond the Royal Gaze: Clanship and Public Healing in Buganda* (Charlottesville, 2010), pp. 149–154.

24. TNA CO 822/812.

25. See especially: S. R. Karugire, *A Political History of Uganda* (Kampala, 2010); P. Mutibwa, *The Buganda Factor in Uganda Politics* (Kampala, 2008); and R. Reid, *A History of Modern Uganda* (Cambridge, 2017).

26. F. Cooper and A. L. Stoler, *Tensions of Empire: Colonial Cultures in a Bourgeois World* (Berkeley and Los Angeles, 1997), pp. vii–viii.

27. S. Heald, *Controlling Anger: The Anthropology of Gisu Violence* (Oxford, 1998), p. 245.

28. P. Khanakwa, 'Masculinity and Nation: Struggles in the Practice of Male Circumcision Among the Bagisu of Eastern Uganda, 1900s to 1960s' (Unpublished PhD thesis, Northwestern University, 2011), pp. 197–204.

29. Ibid., pp. 215–219.

30. Mbale District Archives (MDA) MBL/4/57 (Marriage Customs, Witchcraft), letter from J. Harding Cox, District Medical Officer, Bugisu/Sebei Districts, to Mr. Bwayo, The Administrative Secretary, Bugisu District Administration, 20 August 1964.

31. MDA MBL/4/57, letter from the District Commissioner, Bugisu, to the District Forestry Office, 9 May 1960; Heald, *Controlling Anger*, p. 1.

32. MDA MBL/4/68 (Homicide in Bugisu), 'Minutes of the Security/Intelligence Committee Meeting', 10 August 1964, p. 3.

33. Heald, *Controlling Anger*, pp. 229–230; S. Heald, 'Mafias in Africa: The Rise of Drinking Companies and Vigilante Groups in Bugisu District, Uganda', *Africa* 56 (1986), pp. 446–467.

34. MDA MBL/4/68, F. X. Lubega, District Agricultural Officer, Bugisu/Sebei Districts, 'Increased Agriculture Activity as a Means to Reduce Homicides', 16 June 1965.

35. Interview with Gisu male, approximately 74 years old (MLE-06), Mbale District, 27 October 2011; Interview with Gisu male, approximately 71 years old (MLE-11), Mbale District, 27 October 2011.

36. Interview with Gisu female, approximately 80 years old (MLE-09), Mbale District, 27 October 2011; Interview with Gisu male, approximately 77

years old (MLE-12), Mbale District, 27 October 2011; Interview with Gisu female, approximately 74 years old (MLE-13), Mbale District, 27 October 2011; and Interview with Gisu female, approximately 70 years old (MLE-15), Mbale District, 31 October 2011.

37. Khanakwa, 'Masculinity and Nation', p. 53.

38. Ibid., p. 236. Circumcision year names from 1801–1970 are listed in M. Macpherson, 'Circumcision Year Names (Kamengilo) in Masaba & Their Meanings', *Uganda Journal* 39 (1980), pp. 59–75.

39. Interview with Gisu male, approximately 81 years old (MLE-02), Mbale District, 27 October 2011.

40. Interview with Gisu female, approximately 81 years old (MLE-03), Mbale District, 27 October 2011; Interview with Gisu female, approximately 75 years old (MLE-04), Mbale District, 27 October 2011; Interview with Gisu female, approximately 60 years old (MLE-05), Mbale District, 27 October 2011; Interview MLE-09. On the *basambwa*, see Heald, *Controlling Anger*, p. 205.

41. Interview with Gisu male, approximately 80 years old (MLE-01), Mbale District, 27 October 2011; Interview MLE-03; Interview MLE-04; Interview MLE-05; Interview MLE-06; Interview with Gisu female, approximately 61 years old (MLE-07), Mbale District, 27 October 2011; Interview with Gisu female, approximately 80 years old (MLE-08), Mbale District, 27 October 2011; Interview MLE-12; Interview MLE-13; and Interview with Gisu female, approximately 78 years old (MLE-16), Mbale District, 1 November 2011.

42. Interview MLE-02.

43. Interview MLE-16.

44. Interview MLE-11.

45. Interview MLE-01; Interview MLE-03; Interview MLE-04; Interview MLE-05; Interview MLE-06; Interview MLE-07; Interview MLE-08; Interview MLE-09; Interview with Gisu male, approximately 70 years old (MLE-10), Mbale District, 27 October 2011; Interview MLE-13; Interview MLE-15; Interview MLE-16; and Interview with Gisu male, approximately 77 years old (MLE-18), Mbale District, 1 November 2011.

46. Interview MLE-08; Interview MLE-10; Interview MLE-12; Interview MLE-15; Interview MLE-16; Interview MLE-18.

47. J. La Fontaine, *The Gisu of Uganda* (London, 1959), p. 50; J. La Fontaine, 'Witchcraft in Bugisu', in J. Middleton and E. H. Winter, eds., *Witchcraft and Sorcery in East Africa* (London, 1963), p. 191, fn. 1.

48. Interview MLE-12.

49. Heald, *Controlling Anger*, p. 129.

50. Interview with Gisu female, approximately 70 years old (MLE-15), Mbale District, 31 October 2011.

51. Interview MLE-05.
52. Interview MLE-04.
53. Interview with Gisu male, approximately 71 years old (MLE-11), Mbale District, 27 October 2011.
54. Interview MLE-17.
55. Interview MLE-04; Interview MLE-15; Interview MLE-18.
56. Interview MLE-12.
57. Interview MLE-17.
58. Interview MLE-07. On nuclear test sites, see J. Allman, 'Nuclear Imperialism and the Pan-African Struggle for Peace and Freedom: Ghana, 1959–1962', *Souls* 10(2) (2008), pp. 83–102.
59. Interview MLE-02.
60. Rankin and Philip, 'An Epidemic of Laughing', p. 168.
61. Interview MLE-02.
62. M. Graboyes, *The Experiment Must Continue: Medical Research and Ethics in East Africa, 1940–2014* (Athens, OH, 2015); L. White, *Speaking with Vampires: Rumor and History in Colonial Africa* (Berkeley, 2000).
63. Interview MLE-02.
64. Kagwa, 'The Problem of Mass Hysteria', p. 560.
65. B. H. Kagwa, *A Ugandan: Defiant and Triumphant* (Hicksville, 1978), p. 17. On Kagwa's return, see also 'Dr. Kagwa Home—For Ever', *Uganda Argus*, 23 August 1963, p. 3.
66. Kagwa, *A Ugandan*, p. 130.
67. Ibid., p. 138.
68. Ibid.
69. Ibid., pp. 147–148. On (white) doctor memoirs of Africa, see especially: Vaughan, *Curing Their Ills*, Ch. 7.
70. Kagwa, *A Ugandan*, p. 138.
71. Ibid.
72. Ibid., p. 133.
73. Ibid.
74. Kagwa, 'The Problem of Mass Hysteria', p. 560.
75. Ibid., p. 561.
76. Ibid.
77. Ibid., p. 560.
78. A. P. Noyes and L. C. Kolb, *Modern Clinical Psychiatry*, 6th ed. (Philadelphia, 1963), pp. 430–436.
79. Kagwa, 'The Problem of Mass Hysteria', p. 565.
80. Ibid.
81. Ibid.
82. Rankin and Philip, 'An Epidemic of Laughing', p. 170.

83. Kagwa quoted from J. C. Carothers, *The African Mind in Health and Disease: A Study in Ethnopsychiatry* (Geneva, 1952).
84. Kagwa, 'The Problem of Mass Hysteria', p. 565.
85. On T. A. Lambo, see especially M. M. Heaton, *Black Skin, White Coats: Nigerian Psychiatrists, Decolonization, and the Globalization of Psychiatry* (Ohio, 2013).
86. World Health Organization, *WHO and Mental Health 1949–1961* (Geneva, 1962), p. 34.
87. Kagwa, 'The Problem of Mass Hysteria', p. 562.
88. Ibid., p. 565.
89. Ibid., pp. 562–563.
90. See, for example, 'Epidemic Hysteria', *British Medical Journal*, November 1966, p. 1280; G. Rosen, 'Psychopathology in the Social Process: I. A Study of the Persecution of Witches in Europe as a Contribution to the Understanding of Mass Delusions and Psychic Epidemics', *Journal of Health and Human Behaviour* 3 (1960), pp. 200–211; and F. K. Taylor and R. C. A. Hunter, 'Observation of a Hysterical Epidemic in a Hospital Ward', *Psychiatric Quarterly* 32 (1958), pp. 821–839.
91. R. E. Bartholomew, 'Tarantism, Dancing Mania and Demonopathy: The Anthro-Political Aspects of "Mass Psychogenic Illness"', *Psychological Medicine* 24 (1994), pp. 281–307.
92. Rankin and Philip, 'An Epidemic of Laughing', p. 167.
93. B. H. Kagwa, 'Observations on the Prevalence and Types of Mental Diseases in East Africa', *East African Medical Journal* 42 (1965), p. 673.
94. ACMM, Uganda Government, 'Ministry of Health Annual Report for the Year from 1st July 1963 to 30th June 1964', typescript, 1964, pp. 16, 23.
95. Kagwa, 'The Problem of Mass Hysteria', p. 561.
96. Ibid., pp. 561–562.
97. La Fontaine, *The Gisu*, p. 53.
98. S. R. Whyte, 'Penicillin, Battery Acid and Sacrifice', *Social Science and Medicine* 16 (1982), pp. 2055–2064.
99. Interview MLE-11.
100. Ibid.
101. Interview MLE-01; Interview MLE-02. For fuller treatment of the types of ritual specialists among the Bagisu, see La Fontaine, 'Witchcraft in Bugisu', p. 190.
102. Interview MLE-03; Interview MLE-04.
103. Interview MLE-08; Interview MLE-09; Interview MLE-18.
104. Interview MLE-05.

105. Interview MLE-13; Interview MLE-16; Interview MLE-01; Interview MLE-02; Interview MLE-10; Interview MLE-12.
106. Interview MLE-18.
107. White, *Speaking with Vampires*, Ch. 3.
108. Interview MLE-12.
109. S. Feierman, 'Change in African Therapeutic Systems', *Social Science and Medicine* 13B (1979), pp. 227–284; J. Janzen, *The Quest for Therapy: Medical Pluralism in Lower Zaire* (Berkeley, 1978).
110. J. Orley, 'Indigenous Concepts of Disease and Their Interaction with Scientific Medicine', in E. E. Sabben-Clare, D. J. Bradley, and K. Kirkwood, eds., *Health in Tropical Africa During the Colonial Period: Based on the Proceedings of a Symposium Held at New College, Oxford, 21–23 March 1977* (Oxford, 1980), p. 127; J. C. Ssekemwa gives some examples of this in 'Witchcraft in Buganda Today', *Transition* 30 (1967), pp. 30–39.
111. Interview MLE-07.
112. Heaton, *Black Skin, White Coats*, p. 71.
113. J. B. Loudon, 'Social Aspects of Ideas About Treatment', in A. V. S. de Reuck and Ruth Porter, eds., *Transcultural Psychiatry* (London, 1965).
114. T. A. Lambo, as cited in Loudon, 'Social Aspects of Ideas About Treatment', pp. 192–193.
115. B. Bernstein, 'Social Class, Speech Systems and Psycho-Therapy', *The British Journal of Sociology* 15(1) (1964), pp. 54–64.

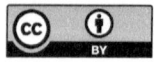

CHAPTER 5

The Psychiatry of Poverty

Addressing a meeting of twenty-five psychiatrists from nine African countries, the UK and the USA at Makerere University College in April 1969, G. Allen German, Professor of Psychiatry, declared that the 'major feature distinguishing psychiatry in Africa from psychiatry in the Western world is poverty'.[1] Poverty and 'associated ignorance' determined 'many of the peculiarities of clinical states', resulted in inadequate treatment facilities, and interfered both with the use of facilities by patients and with patient follow-up. For German, the 'psychiatry of poverty' entailed a focus not on the types of disorders patients might suffer as a result of poverty, but the ways in which an understanding of poverty might determine the development of mental health services in a particular context. Due to constraints on resources and a lack of manpower in many African contexts, he contended, efforts to develop mental health services needed to focus on the training of non-psychiatrists, whether psychiatric nurses, psychiatric social workers (PSWs), or psychiatric clinical officers. These 'psychiatric auxiliaries' were not only more likely to be drawn from the same areas as their patients, and so speak their languages, but could be trained to take on some of the responsibility for mental health care at minimal cost.[2]

Arguments for the rapid expansion of psychiatry in the late 1960s and early 1970s appeared entirely logical in light of research within trans-cultural psychiatry and psychiatric epidemiology that was suggesting that the overall incidence and clinical picture of mental illness in Africa

© The Author(s) 2019
Y. Pringle, *Psychiatry and Decolonisation in Uganda*,
Mental Health in Historical Perspective,
https://doi.org/10.1057/978-1-137-60095-0_5

was little different from that elsewhere in the world. If anything, pressure on already overstretched psychiatric institutions would only grow in coming years, as urbanisation and other social changes made it more difficult for the mentally ill to be cared for by their families. Like psychiatrists elsewhere in Africa, Uganda's psychiatrists actively contributed to this increasingly transnational and global body of knowledge that was not only challenging many of the earlier assumptions of colonial psychiatrists, but also promising findings that were relevant to changing social and economic circumstances.[3] One such collaborative study between German and M. I. Assael, an Israeli psychiatrist, along with J. M. Namboze, Uganda's first female doctor, and F. J. Bennett, of the Department of Preventive Medicine, Makerere Medical School, found that among 100 expectant mothers, depressive reactions were common, something 'in keeping with the recent realization that depression is a frequent disorder in the rural African'.[4] Presenting the results of a study of two hundred and sixty-three pregnant Ugandan women, John Cox similarly argued that the myth that African women were free from emotional disorders during pregnancy was unsubstantiated. Instead, he found similar rates of women with pronounced psychiatric symptoms in Uganda to those reported from studies of European and American women.[5] H. G. Egdell's research on child psychiatry, meanwhile, was crucial in helping to establish child psychiatry as a serious area of study outside of Europe and the USA. Egdell stressed the similarities in the clinical picture of child neurology with the limited studies already conducted in the USA, India and Nigeria, and made practical suggestions for the development of services for children in developing countries.[6]

By the early 1970s, research by psychiatrists from across developing countries was sufficient to prompt *The British Journal of Psychiatry* to commission a series of review articles: Carlos A. Leon on psychiatry in Latin America, J. S. Neki on psychiatry in South-East Asia and German on psychiatry in sub-Saharan Africa.[7] Published in 1972, German's article synthesised two decades of research by African and expatriate psychiatrists that overwhelmingly showed the fallacies of research by colonial psychiatrists. While he noted serious problems with the methodology of some studies, the overwhelming picture of psychiatry in Africa was that of similarity to other parts of the world. The prevalence of mental illness 'seems much the same as elsewhere', he noted: 'schizophrenia, manic-depressive disorder and organic psychoses exist in their familiar forms, although in different proportions; neurotic illness is widespread, although little studied;

psychogeriatric problems are beginning to appear'.[8] Where there were differences, they were mainly in behaviour and personality changes, as well as the emphasis placed on physical, as opposed to psychological symptoms. Rather than reflecting racial difference, then, the clinical picture of mental illness seemed to be determined by 'physiological deprivations and physical disease' as well as 'cultural differences and widespread illiteracy'.[9] As a body of evidence, such ideas about mental illness suggested that provision for the mentally ill in existing mental hospitals was inadequate, but offered no easy answers as to how far psychiatry in developing countries should differ from that in Europe and the USA. Rather, it highlighted the potential strain being placed on a small number of trained psychiatrists, which was only likely to increase in the future. As G. M. Carstairs, President of the World Federation for Mental Health (WFMH), stressed in 1972, what was clear, was that as 'the presence of psychiatric morbidity becomes more apparent' in developing countries, so 'the limitations of medically-trained manpower also come to be recognized'.[10]

The transnational and global context of research was crucial in stimulating the reorganisation of psychiatric services in Uganda. Yet the direction this took, and the ability of psychiatrists to effect change, cannot be separated from the political context of development and nation building. In Uganda, the colonial government had since the Second World War pursued 'development' largely through the 'modernising' projects of state-led industrialisation and the diversification of the agricultural sector.[11] After Independence in 1962, the Uganda Government, under Milton Obote, similarly prioritised industrialisation, but with a much keener sense of the need to overcome the inequitable distribution of wealth and power, particularly between urban and rural areas. Here, the differences were stark: between 1960–1969, peasants in remote rural areas earned approximately 305–355 shillings a year, 1% of that of a senior civil servant, and five times less than the average worker in Buganda, in central Uganda.[12] While the Uganda Government did little to address high government wages, they aimed to combat poverty through an ambitious expansion of social, educational, medical and health services through the 1960s.[13] *The First Five-Year Development Plan* (1962) spoke of their intention 'to develop educational facilities on such a scale and in such a way as to provide for every child, regardless of the social or economic circumstances of parents', and 'to provide a comprehensive national health service available to all citizens regardless of means'.[14] The investment needed to develop services in such a way was prohibitive, however, not only financially, but also logistically, as increasing demand for medical and health services strained manpower resources. Pressure on services in urban centres, too, similarly grew as Ugandans flocked to the towns following Independence, putting further constraints on rural development plans.[15] Here, psychiatry was just one voice at a time when multiple different services were competing for centrality within the development priorities of the nation. Addressing the same meeting of psychiatrists at Makerere at which German had articulated the 'psychiatry of poverty', the Deputy Minister of Health, S. W. Uringi, asked if it was possible 'to so modify traditional psychiatric activity that, by making use of resources which are available in developing populations, adequate services can be provided more cheaply than has been the case in the past?'[16] Declaring mental hospitals to be an expensive means of keeping people out of sight, he urged psychiatrists to consider other ways of deploying psychiatric personnel: 'What level of training do they require? What facilities do they need? What resources already exist in the community which can be utilised and adapted to minimise expenditure?'[17]

During the late 1960s and early 1970s, psychiatry flourished in a period of experimentation and innovation intended to extend the reach of psychiatry at minimal cost. Uganda's psychiatrists established a Mental Health Advisory Committee (MHAC) with the aim of advising the Ministry of Health on policy and lobbying for reform. They discussed and trialled proposals to train PSWs, interpreters and psychiatric clinical workers, and to establish mental health clinics in hospitals where responsibility would be delegated to non-specialists. Recognising that they needed not only to persuade government officials, but other professionals—health, legal and welfare—of the need to take an interest in mental health, they combined pilot schemes with mental health education programmes. They set up Africa's first National Association for Mental Health (the NAMH), launched training courses for police officers, lawyers and health workers in hospitals outside of Kampala and participated in a television series entitled 'The Sick Mind'. These activities aimed not only at spreading Western ideas about mental illness to the wider Ugandan public, but to mobilise supportive professionals in order to extend the reach of psychiatry beyond that which could have been achieved by psychiatrists alone.

This period of relative political stability in Uganda's history since 1962 was one of a new contextually sensitive politics, and it was one that demanded the refiguring of the relationship not only between psychiatrists and patients, but also between psychiatry and other institutions and services. The newly independent Uganda Government was accountable to its citizens in ways that the colonial government never had been, and psychiatrists were well aware of the need to demonstrate the relevance of their work. In this, many of Uganda's psychiatrists benefitted from their association with Makerere Medical School, which during the 1960s became an internationally renowned centre of research and practice, attracting over £280,000 in medical research grants between 1964–1967 (approximately 5 million pounds in today's terms).[18] Yet psychiatry nevertheless faced ongoing practical constraints on its ability to translate rhetoric and small-scale experiments into real, felt change 'on the ground'. Much of this was beyond the control of the psychiatrists. Indeed, it proved impossible, logistically and financially, to train sufficient specialist personnel in such a short period of time. Similarly, the scale of the task of moving psychiatry away from a system that continued to bring only the most 'urgent' or violent patients to the gates of Butabika Hospital was overwhelming. But equally, the limits to reform might be best understood as a failure to fully consider the needs and priorities of the patients themselves.

PROBLEMS OF SOCIAL AND ECONOMIC CHANGE

Research in the field of mental health may have formed part of a broad transnational endeavour to show that the clinical picture of mental illness was little different in Africa to that elsewhere, but much of it was driven by concern about two key features of social and economic change in early postcolonial Uganda: education and urbanisation. Education provision had expanded rapidly in the final years of colonial rule, with double the number of pupils attending primary school and eight times the number of students in secondary education by 1962.[19] Expansion continued through the 1960s, with education positioned as essential not only for economic growth, but also for the well-being of the nation.[20] Urbanisation, too, accelerated across East Africa after Independence, as rural migrants moved to cities in search of work, adding to the growth of an informal sector and posing challenges to municipal order.[21] These changes brought students and urban residents to the forefront of psychiatric attention and provided an important way of demonstrating the relevance of psychiatry in a new sociopolitical context. As Bennett explained in 1967, students at Makerere faced a series of unique stresses.

'The majority', he noted, 'are the first generation of the educated. Great expectations rest upon their shoulders. For most, arrival at Makerere means a sudden change from a traditional, family centred way of life to the novel freedoms and restraints of a European patterned centre of learning set in the forefront of the intellectual, political and technological revolution of mid-20th century Africa'.[22]

In 1969, German, together with O. P. Arya, of the Department of Preventive Medicine, undertook a study of psychiatric morbidity among students at Makerere University College. 'This student population', they noted, 'is of peculiar interest to psychiatrists, partly because it is predominantly African, but also because these African undergraduates occupy a central position in the whirl of social and cultural changes sweeping across East Africa'.[23] While German and Arya found no evidence to suggest that mental illness was on the increase at Makerere, they argued that the rate of mental breakdown was relatively high: of 1112 attendees to the Student Health Service, 121 (10.8%) were found to be suffering from a psychiatric disorder—mostly anxiety and depression.[24] Students reported overwhelming stress relating to examinations and study, fears of having contracted venereal disease, as well as anxiety about the size and potency of their genitals (the last two perhaps unsurprising given the high incidence of gonorrhoea on campus).[25] Yet among these students, at least two were surprised that their accounts of their emotions, which included feelings of worthless and suicidal ideas, had led them to be referred to a psychiatrist for depression.[26]

Research on student mental health reinforced wider concerns about the effects of the expansion of education through the 1960s. This was not because it was believed that the stresses of 'western' education in itself would in some way lead to mental breakdown, however. Indeed, in this way, the research in Uganda differed from that of Raymond Prince on 'brain-fag syndrome' among unmarried adult Nigerian males studying in England. This constellation of complaints, which was marked by 'intellectual impairment, sensory impairment (chiefly visual), and somatic complaints most commonly of pain or burning in the head and neck', was, Prince hypothesised, 'in some way related to the imposition of European learning techniques upon the Nigerian personality'.[27] Instead, German and Arya offered a social and psychological explanation for the relatively high rates of mental illness seen among East African students. For them, it was unsurprising that students might break down while studying, given 'the enormous emphasis placed on academic success by families and society'.[28]

The social aspects of urbanisation were similarly stressed by research-ers who looked towards the growing number of migrants moving to Kampala—often living alone and in poverty.[29] Many came from rural areas, contributing to an increase in population in Buganda of approx-imately 40% between 1949 and 1958. But one of the most striking features of Uganda was the high level of international migration from neighbouring African countries, comprising approximately 10% of the population by the early 1960s.[30] Immigrants from Rwanda, who were increasingly moving away from the border area in south-west Uganda in search of employment opportunities, were of particular concern: by 1966, Rwandan immigrants comprised approximately 4.5% of the pop-ulation of Kampala, with many having first entered Uganda during the 1959–1964 Tutsi refugee crisis.[31] Rwandans were also the fastest grow-ing group of inpatients at Butabika Hospital, comprising over 10% of first admissions in the first half of 1968.[32]

Despite the refugee background of some of these immigrants, no link was made between violence and psychological health. Indeed, as we shall see in Chapter 7, the notion that refugees might have unique men-tal and psychological needs as a result of their exposure to violence, and ongoing uncertainty about their futures, was rarely considered in Africa before the 1980s. Instead, as Bennett and Assael contended in 1970, their presence in the psychiatric system was due to a 'changing society' that not only made mental health problems more visible, but was leaving increasing numbers of individuals without adequate social support networks. As one Rwandan living near Kampala commented, while he had not been rejected by his neighbours, he still felt isolated: 'No-one will help if something hap-pened'. In a comment that points to disconnects between expectations and reality, another complained: 'I am disappointed with friendship here where no one will help unless you pay – this is not Rwanda'.[33] Bennett and Assael reported finding high levels of alcoholism, depression and anti-so-cial behaviour among the Rwandan immigrants they studied living near Kasangati Health Centre. Yet it was immigrant children for whom they expressed the most concern. In addition to having parents 'caught in a web of depression, alcoholism and isolation', school—'the one institution which would help in fitting them into the new society'—was out of reach due to the inability of their parents to pay fees. If support measures were not set in place, they added, 'A frustrated and delinquent second generation might evolve'.[34]

Psychiatric research presented a coherent view of how social and economic changes were shaping present and future mental health needs. But the voices and opinions of those under the psychiatric gaze were obscured within it, not only in terms of descriptions of their symptoms, but whether their problems were psychiatric or social in nature, and how they might best be helped. The comments of the two students who were 'surprised' at being diagnosed with depression hint at this. But undergraduate students at Makerere in particular had their own ideas about the problems of education. They were, for example, acutely aware of their isolation on the campus at Makerere University College which, despite being located on the edge of Kampala, was 'still basically a community fenced in, with a gate guarded day and night, an appearance of social exclusiveness'.[35] The weight of the institution and its expectations also weighed heavily on their minds, not only as a result of the lengthy 'filtering process' of national examinations that had selected them as an elite group, but through the way the institution unwittingly forced students to choose between 'the West' and their cultural roots.[36] As Peter Nazareth, Ugandan literary critic and Makerere graduate recalled: 'There was a heavy colonial pall over the place which made it quite hard to be creative instead of imitative, to challenge any of the norms. I mean, we were supposedly the elite who had made it up there and yet somehow there was this feeling that we were not good enough. We were not European'.[37] While the curriculum was changing during the 1960s, with increased recognition of the importance of African history and literature, among other subjects, Makerere as an institution was still heavily Europeanised.[38] Much of this found expression in East African literature during the 1960s and 1970s. The journalist-protagonist of John Nagenda's 'And This, At Last', written while an undergraduate, is a product of a colonial school education and demonstrates a condescending attitude towards village life. Yet after interviewing an old man, his superficiality is shattered: the journalist and fellow graduates are 'doomed to sterility and civilization'.[39] In Jonathan Kariara's poem, 'The Dream of Africa', moreover, similarly written while at Makerere, Kariara described how the 'white clay of foreign education' was 'stifling' the African. Critiquing the cultural dependency created by education (and indeed medicine), Kariara wrote of the anxieties arising from what was essentially a reworking of the self:

Doctor, what ails me, what ails -
(The bottled ale I took the other night to forget)
The ready-made pill prescription
For a slight mental maladjustment
Due to...due to...that's not for us to know:
It is the knowing doctor's secret.
"Business, you see."
So we glibly take it, the pill,
Which smoothes the pain and smoothes the nerves,
And sends the disease to sleep.

Even then, despite all expectations, there was no guarantee that this preparation was not all for nothing when the 'white clay' was removed: 'Will it be the pearl in the oyster shell, / Or mere rottenness?'[40] These Makerere graduates would have agreed with the psychiatrists that it was not 'education' per se that was a problem, but would likely have had very different ideas about the nature of changes required. Rather than seeing their experiences as indicative of the need for an increase in the capacity of mental health services in Uganda, it was the approaches, values and content of education that needed to be addressed.

Analysis of the problems facing students and urban migrants pointed to a need for wide-ranging reforms not only within education, but in the provision of social welfare services. Yet psychiatry's interest in these groups did not translate into additional, targeted psychiatric support. While from 1966 psychiatrists ran a monthly clinic at Kasangati Health Centre, an area with a relatively high number of migrants, as well as individuals living alone, there was no specific service for Rwandan immigrants, and no psychiatrist who could speak Kinyarwanda.[41] At Makerere, too, students seeking assistance for anxiety and depression continued to rely on the Student Health Service which, reflecting the insular nature of the campus, was used by an estimated 80–90% of all students in any one year.[42] The medical practitioners who staffed the service had no specialist training in mental health, their main role in these cases being to counsel students. The small number of students who showed signs of schizophrenia or psychosis were referred to a psychiatrist at Mulago Hospital, but otherwise mental health was handled internally, and there were no plans to increase or change this service.[43] The importance of concern about education and urbanisation should instead be located in the way it provided a bridge between psychiatry and the needs and priorities of the developmentalist state—a way of demonstrating psychiatry's relevance to both state and society. In an attempt to combat the long-standing neglect of psychiatry by government officials, the psychiatrists of the late 1960s and early 1970s would use it to point to signs of growing pressure on medical, health and social welfare services in the future.

PSYCHIATRY AND THE DEVELOPMENT OF HEALTH SERVICES

Like many other African countries, Uganda inherited a health system from the British in which care was concentrated in large, predominantly urban hospitals. The expense required to maintain this health system was staggering, constituting as much as 70% of government expenditure in the years between Independence in 1962 and Idi Amin's coup in 1971.[44] Instead of focusing on the development of basic health services, the newly independent Ministry of Health maintained this highly centralised system, prioritising the expansion of central referral hospitals (including the completion of Butabika Hospital and a state-of-the-art New Mulago Hospital), then district hospitals and, on a much smaller scale, rural health clinics.[45] The high capital expenditure required by this development strategy went against World Bank policy (which Uganda abandoned in 1964) and was subject to fierce criticism by medical practitioners, but it pleased voters and their demands for more hospitals. 'The cry by every Ugandan', Minister of Health Emmanuel Lumu exclaimed in 1970, is 'more hospitals, more dispensaries, more aid posts, more medicine and so on'. But, he added, 'I am afraid that we cannot keep up with the demands of the country'.[46] Rural populations continued to be under-served, not least by psychiatry, where there were still few specialist personnel and the mental health services in Kampala were remote.

The MHAC, established in early 1967 by German, set itself an ambitious goal: they aimed to convince the Ministry of Health to aim for mental health to comprise 25–30% of the national medical effort at all levels—beds, staffing and budget. This figure presupposed a growing need in the coming years as investments in public health and preventive medicine reduced rates of physical illness and made mental illness more visible. While they could not claim that voters were demanding new psychiatric services, they argued that the pressures brought on by education and urbanisation, as well as the 'increasing burdens of responsibility' placed on the workforce, was 'accelerating the demand for psychiatric treatment many times over'.[47] Above all, the MHAC wanted to overcome the lack of investment and interest in psychiatry since the colonial period. In line with more general investment in district hospitals, the Ministry of Health had made provisions for eight 16-bed psychiatric units in their *Second Five-Year Development Plan* (1966), but the MHAC saw this as a potential 'embarrassment to the psychiatric services'. In an official statement to the Ministry of Health in 1967, the MHAC expressed their dissatisfaction, arguing that 62-bed units with outpatient facilities, and staffed by a doctor and 'a proper psychiatric team' of nurses and social workers, were instead necessary to meet growing demand. While in the past 'priorities in the field of mental health have been overlooked', the MHAC hoped that things would soon be remedied.[48]

The MHAC represented an official collaboration between psychiatrists employed by Makerere University College and those employed by the Uganda Government. Sanctioned by the Ministry of Health, this advisory body comprised of Ugandan and expatriate psychiatrists, as well as other individuals with an interest in the development of mental health services.[49] While in 1967 the MHAC was small, consisting of German, Stephen B. Bosa, James F. Wood, and a medical officer, mental nurse and matron attached to Butabika Hospital, by 1971 it had expanded to include psychiatrists, mental nurses, a high court judge, a police commissioner and members of the Ministry of Health.[50] The MHAC worked closely to advise and implement new plans for the extension of mental health services, lobbying the Ministry of Health for financial support, when necessary. Members of the MHAC also investigated and prepared papers on a range of topics, opening up a dialogue between psychiatrists and the Ministry of Health on such themes as interpreters and the Uganda Psychiatric Service, psychiatric social work and trial mental health clinics at Jinja and Mbarara Hospitals.[51] The discussions highlighted a range of opinions and suggestions as to what should take priority, yet all aimed at extending the reach of psychiatry at a time of increasing pressure on government finances.

Despite their ambitious goals, the MHAC experienced many of the same frustrations that Bosa had earlier in the decade when he had approached the Ministry of Health with suggestions for reform. One of the earliest proposals to meet with failure was that for an official cadre of interpreters in psychiatric service. A briefing note written by Egdell described the language barrier that was preventing adequate communication between patients and staff, as well as contributing to an 'unpleasant isolation' of many inpatients. Highlighting the contingent nature of psychiatry, Egdell noted that 'Without an interpreter the psychiatrist is in the same position as a blind physician, unable to see physical signs'.[52] Beyond English, Luganda and Swahili, knowledge of most of Uganda's fifty-plus languages was almost non-existent among expatriate and Ugandan psychiatrists, ward sisters, PSWs and medical students who, coming from across East Africa, 'often cannot even speak Luganda'.[53] The ability of nursing staff to converse at a basic level was not enough, as Egdell stressed: 'We need precise details of subtle changes in thinking, feeling and behaviour which are often expressed in African languages with the greatest difficulty'.[54] The MHAC therefore proposed to the Ministry of Health that an initial group of twenty-five interpreters be trained to cover Mulago and Butabika Hospitals, psychiatric social work, social and occupational therapy, and the courts. Within a year, however, the plan was dropped. In addition to the administrative difficulties of introducing a new cadre of staff at a time when the Uganda Government was streamlining the civil service, there were questions of cost, training and delegation. The interpreters would require 'an understanding of psychiatric, psychological and medical terminology in English and the other languages mentioned above, appreciating the significance of these terms in relation to indigenous languages and customs', yet who could ensure their accuracy?[55]

The inflexibility of the Ministry of Health was again seen in response to plans to train a new cadre of PSWs. A two-year scheme proposed by Bosa and F. J. Harris, World Health Organization (WHO)-supported Lecturer in Psychiatric Social Work, the proposal was intended as a way of bolstering follow-up and family outreach in district hospitals. PSWs would take social histories from patients and relatives, explain diagnoses and methods of treatment, prepare families to receive patients after discharge and be responsible for after-care, counselling of parents and mental health education in rural communities. These duties were 'arduous and time-consuming' but considered necessary to ensure the functioning of psychiatry beyond Butabika and Mulago Hospitals.[56] With financial support from Makerere, Harris started training a small number of PSWs, but the Ministry of Health refused to recognise the Diploma in Psychiatric Social Work. Just as with the interpreters in psychiatric service, this new cadre required the creation of a new position within the civil service, and with it, new administrative and financial obligations.

With a Ministry of Health that was reluctant to commit to large, potentially costly schemes, the MHAC focused on small pilot projects, funded jointly by Makerere and the Ministry of Health, and aimed at exploring how mental health services could be best developed at minimal cost. In 1968, E. B. Ssekabembe launched a Jinja Mental Health Follow-up Clinic trial, to operate every last Friday of the month.[57] In the first few months of operation, between 5 and 11 patients attended the clinic each month and received medication on an outpatient basis, including sedatives (such as Largactil) and anticonvulsants (such as Phenobarb). Yet with Jinja Hospital failing to release a medical officer (MO) to assist Ssekabembe once a month, it proved impossible to train anyone to take over the clinic. Added to this were medical assistants at Butabika Hospital who had 'forgotten' to advertise the clinic. Reflecting a recurring gap between intentions and the ability to transform practices and behaviours, one patient complained that the clinic had not been well advertised at all, and pointed to over 20 cases in his village, near Jinja, who were in need of help.[58] Demand for a clinic was also evident in a trial at Mbarara Hospital, which Bosa operated once a month, hoping that 'perhaps with luck one might stimulate enough interest in some doctors for them to devote more attention to the understanding and care of the mentally sick'. Between 14 and 24 patients attended each month in the first six months, with one MO, B. Kahigwa, requesting further training at so he could take over the running of the clinic. Despite similar problems in advertising their work beyond a small area around the hospital, Bosa called the trial a resounding success: not only had it reduced the number of referrals and readmissions to Butabika Hospital, but the 'physical appearance of a consultant psychiatrist at the hospital helped to improve the attitude towards mental illness, management and treatment in both staff and patients, and also in the general community'.[59] In the coming months, Bosa added, he was confident he could 'demonstrate convincingly (with figures)' that Ministry of Health investment in mental health at Mbarara 'is now essential and very urgently required'.[60] Well aware from his own previous experiences of the difficulties of persuading government administrators for support, Bosa knew he not only had to draw up a careful case for funding and personnel, but be wary of how he presented any practical difficulties experienced.

While the pilot mental health clinics, operating every four to six weeks, did not represent a huge time commitment in and of themselves, they nevertheless required seemingly endless energy from those involved.

After a full week's research, teaching and clinical duties, German would on a Friday once a month drive to Soroti, 300 miles north-east of Kampala, check into a hotel and be ready for work at a mental health clinic at Soroti Hospital by seven o'clock the following morning. On the Sunday, German would then devote three to four hours delivering a case conference and lecture series to senior nursing staff, MOs and any other interested parties, before driving back to Kampala. Bosa, too, would travel to Mbarara and other district hospitals after a full week's work, dedicating his Saturdays to clinical work, court work and the training of medical and health workers.[61] In addition to the personal drain of this work, there was ongoing frustration at the slow pace of change, as well as fears that activities that took staff away from Butabika Hospital were contributing to an increasing reliance there on psychotropic drugs.[62] Indeed, despite the relatively large number of psychiatrists in Uganda in the late 1960s and early 1970s, pressures on time meant few practical changes to conditions at Butabika Hospital. As John Orley noted: 'Doctors in a hospital admitting over 60 patients a week, and who usually do not speak the patient's language find it almost impossible to do more than give rough symptomatic treatment with medication and E.C.T., and sometimes do not bother with the niceties of diagnosis'.[63] By the end of 1968, Bosa had decided to relinquish his research and teaching responsibilities at Makerere and to return to primarily clinical work, stressing that he 'would have better immediate opportunities to utilize my potential abilities' at Butabika Hospital.[64]

The early experiences and setbacks faced by the MHAC made it clear that while increased investment, improved facilities, and new specialist training programmes was the ideal, financial and administrative constraints meant they could only work with existing resources, of which 'manpower', as it was called, was considered to be the most valuable.[65] Training new psychiatrists was not only costly but also time-consuming, offering little chance of expanding psychiatry in the short term. Medical assistants, on the other hand, already existed in relatively large numbers, being regarded as the front line of health care provision in rural areas.[66] Based on his observations at Soroti, German estimated that one in five psychiatric cases went in the first instance to general hospital outpatient clinics, where they were attended to by medical assistants.[67] In district hospitals, according to Egdell, medical assistants took on work with inpatients that was similar to that of an intern: 'Histories are taken and initial provisional diagnosis [sic.] are made'.[68] It was in outpatient departments and rural dispensaries that their value was truly felt, however. There, they saw all patients in the first instance, selecting from them five per cent who needed to be seen by an MO. 'The remaining 95%', Egdell noted, 'are independently diagnosed and treated by the medical assistant himself'.[69] In rural dispensaries, moreover, medical assistants were in sole charge, overseeing 25–30 inpatient beds, in addition to fifty or more outpatients a day. As such, they represented untapped potential for mental health care. '[The] medical assistant fully trained in psychiatry', Egdell stressed, 'would become a member of the psychiatric team up-country or possibly in the national mental hospital. Whilst continuing in their traditional role as equivalent to house officer or intern, they would also provide continuity in psychiatric leadership in the inevitable absences of the psychiatrist'.[70]

The training of medical assistants in psychiatry was not uncontroversial. Concerns were raised, for example, that while medical assistants saw hundreds of patients every day in outpatient departments and dispensaries, requiring them to be on the lookout for cases of mental illness would potentially 'put too much load' on them. While most patients would likely be non-violent, personal safety would also need to be considered, as too would the implications for the profession of assistants taking on sole responsibility for both diagnosis and treatment.[71] Despite these concerns, 'there was unanimity' among the MHAC 'that some form of training should be given to medical assistants'.[72] Bosa and Ssekabembe provided a small amount of informal in-service training in psychiatry to medical assistants in district hospitals during their visits, highlighting their value in being able to speak patients' languages and understand local cultural idioms of madness.[73] In June 1969, moreover, German, J. W. S. Kasirye, Bosa, Wood, Assael, and Ssekabembe submitted a memo to the Ministry of Health setting out potential options for the training of medical assistants in psychiatry, including an eight-week practical course based at Butabika Hospital. 'With appropriate training', it was hoped, the medical assistant would be able to diagnose patients, the majority of whom presented only 'with vague somatic complaints', and in many instances treat them successfully.[74] The proposal, meeting the Ministry of Health's position that any changes require minimal administrative or financial implications, was accepted by the Uganda Government and Makerere University College. By 1971, medical assistants were receiving 'comprehensive teaching in basic psychology' in the first year of their training, and plans were underway to include clinical psychiatry in the second and third years.[75] This model of training and delegating responsibility would come to be recognised internationally as the defining feature of psychiatry in Uganda.

MENTAL HEALTH EDUCATION

With the number of trained medical assistants remaining small until well into the 1970s, and the number of PSWs almost non-existent, in most areas there was still almost no outpatient or after-care available for those seeking relief from mental distress. One nurse who worked at Kabale Hospital, in south-western Uganda, in the late 1960s and early 1970s, described her frustration at the limited assistance they could provide to patients who came to their doors. While the hospital did at times have a small supply of Largactil, it was kept in a locked box, closely guarded by the sole doctor who had been trained to dispense it. With little else to offer, they sent most patients away.[76] The inability of psychiatry to effect widespread, practical reforms in the short term also meant little change to admission patterns at Butabika Hospital. As under colonial rule, violence remained a recurring reason for admission, being the main cause in approximately half of all cases in 1968.[77] Pressures on time, as well as difficulties in communication, also meant that diagnoses continued to be made with limited information, and reflected behaviour observed in the period immediately leading up to admission. One man, who had long history of 'behaving and talking strangely and aggressively', had problems sleeping, and so relied on an alcoholic sedative—¼–½ pint of spirit, distilled from banana beer. Rarely violent, his behaviour was suggestive of an underlying psychological disorder, yet when he suddenly became violent, prompting his being taken to Butabika Hospital, he was diagnosed with 'alcoholic confusional state', and treated by sedation with phenothiazines, before being released home shortly after.[78] Also in line with earlier trends, the number of admissions continued to rise at Butabika Hospital, reaching 3036 between July 1967 and June 1968, with pressure on accommodation meaning that most needed to be discharged within eight weeks.[79] The dangers of the increasing pressure to discharge patients without adequate provision for follow-up support were made painfully clear in 1970, when a policeman, recently released from Butabika Hospital and certified fit to return to work, shot dead the Manager of Mwenge Tea Growers Estate in a fit of confusion.[80]

The MHAC were aware of such problems, but unable to train a cadre of psychiatric auxiliaries overnight, they instead stressed the importance of mental health education as a way of mobilising other professionals to fulfil their legal and social responsibilities towards the mentally ill. In light of the colonial legacy linking psychiatry with violence, police officers were given special attention in attempts to reform psychiatry. 'If he is to do his work well in this field', as Wood noted, 'he needs to have some of the skills of the psychiatric social worker, the psychiatric nurse and the psychiatrist'.[81] In a lecture to lawyers, moreover, Wood explained the main symptoms, treatment and legal considerations of personality disorders, as well as illness caused by organic or physical diseases, schizophrenia and manic-depressive psychosis.[82] Reflecting an increasingly dominant trend within transcultural psychiatry, he stressed that mental illness was both universal and shaped by culture, something that had relevance to the interpretation of the law. Hallucinations, he noted, were 'very real to the subject':

> People with spears, lions and snakes come through windows and doors and crowd round him on the bed. He can hear people talking, threatening and abusing him. Such subjects may jump through the window to escape their hallucinatory persecutors or may unfortunately pick up the ever ready panga from below the bed and "defend" themselves. Usually this results only in a chair being chopped up for a lion but occasionally and tragically a child, a father, mother or brother may be standing by the bedside and may be the victim.[83]

Such a description was reminiscent of earlier colonial interest in the content of 'native' delusions, but was framed here in more culturally sensitive terms.

In educating lawyers about mental illness, Wood took on something of a social advisory role, commenting on social problems that he felt could be more effectively dealt with by increased treatment services and possible changes in the handling of the law. Homosexuality was one such issue. In line with psychiatric thinking in Europe and the USA in the late 1960s, Wood defined homosexuality as 'a sexual perversion resulting from a personality disorder'.[84] While psychiatrists in colonial Africa had had little to say on the subject of homosexuality, seeing it, along with transvestitism and paedophilia, as extremely rare,[85] the effects of negative attitudes towards homosexuality had been raised as a problem in more recent research on student mental health.[86] Changing attitudes towards homosexuality, according to Wood, stemmed directly from legislation introduced under colonial rule.[87] The Penal Code criminalised homosexuality as an 'unnatural offence', placing it alongside bestiality. Any person found to have committed the offence could be charged with a felony and be liable for up to seven years in prison.[88] While only a few men were imprisoned under this legislation—one in 1956, four in 1959 and one in 1960, for example—the law was regarded as having potentially long-term ramifications.[89] Referring to 'homosexual acts between consenting adults in private', Wood argued that it would appear that the '(male) homosexual has been debarred from exercising personal liberty in the matter of sexual practice and that such legislation might be seen to contribute to the causation of mental illness in that it directly (and indirectly by influencing social attitudes) increases the psychological stresses the homosexual must overcome'.[90] For Wood, the homosexual was not only suffering from a sexual perversion, but at risk of serious mental illness from outside pressures—from punitive legislation and social attitudes that were shaped by it. While Wood did not explicitly request that lawyers attempt to seek changes in the law, he emphasised that it was only those homosexuals who engaged in sex with minors who should be considered as a serious problem for society, as this 'might tend to mould them also to the same sexual habit'.[91]

Building on the success of such lectures, Wood negotiated funding from the Uganda Government for a training course on mental health for police officers.[92] Wood's topics included a history of psychiatric services in Uganda, the state of contemporary mental health provision, as well as the signs and symptoms of different types of mental illness. Describing a situation that could have been applied to Uganda at any point during the last forty years, he stressed that officers in rural areas 'may have to look after some very sick patients for several days and may have difficulty in getting medical attention for the patient....They may have difficulty coping with excited patients who may tend to become violent....They may have difficulties with patients who refuse food and fluids....They may find that if they put mentally ill patients together without someone to look after them that the patients may harm each other'.[93] Police officers, Wood stressed, had to recognise their vital role in mental health services, not only in identifying whether a person required medical treatment or restraint, but also in acting 'as transporters, minders and providers until the mentally ill person could be safely delivered to Butabika Hospital or to the Mulago Hospital Psychiatric Outpatient Centre'.[94] The police already required many skills usually filled by social services—now 'psychiatric patient management' had to be another.[95]

The 'public' targeted through such seminars and lectures was limited to 'interested' professionals, and they found, time and again, that they were required to fight against a broad 'public apathy' to mental health activities.[96] This was no less the case with responses to the NAMH, founded in 1967 under the leadership of Bosa and German.[97] The NAMH was certainly the first association of its kind in East Africa and appears also to have been the first on the continent.[98] The concept of a mental health association was not completely new: in 1956, Tewfik had established a Mental Hospitals Voluntary Association, which ran with a committee of five Europeans, five Asians and five Africans until Tewfik's departure in 1958.[99] Yet while Tewfik's Association had focused primarily on bringing volunteer visitors into the mental hospital and giving comfort to the mentally ill, the NAMH was concerned with increasing public knowledge about mental health, improving the status of the mentally ill, and developing strategies for its prevention—the NAMH looked to the world outside the mental hospital, rather than in.[100]

The idea for the association had first been proposed by women associated with the medical community on Mulago hill, including Ethel Bosa (Bosa's first wife), Mrs. Kasirye (wife of J. W. S. Kasirye, then Medical Superintendent of Butabika Hospital), Harriet Kibukamusoke (wife of John Kibukamusoke, Professor of Medicine at Mulago Hospital and first African President of the Association of Physicians of East Africa) and Dorothy Wood (Wood's wife and German's sister).[101] Ganda women in particular remained active in the early years of the association, reflecting an upsurge in social and political activism among women in central Uganda during the 1960s.[102] By 1970, membership of the NAMH had reached 90, comprising, in addition to Ganda women, members of the Asian lay public.

For a brief period in the late 1960s and early 1970s, the NAMH was active in commissioning newspaper articles on mental illness for *Taifa Empya*, a Luganda newspaper. These attracted an enthusiastic response from Ugandan supporters of the Association, and by 1970, staff and students at Bishop Tucker College, Mukono, had translated articles into Karamajong, Runyankole and Luo-Lango.[103] Members also organised seminars covering topics such as suicide, alcoholism, homosexuality and stigma.[104] In a seminar entitled 'Suicide and the Law', held in December

1970, Frank Farrelly, Consultant Psychiatrist, Butabika Hospital, presented alongside Justice Fuad, of the High Court, and Bishop Christopher Senyonjo. Fuad's paper, entitled 'Insanity and the Law', highlighted how while attempted suicide was still an offence in Uganda, the High Court had 'attempted to discourage prosecutions'.[105] Citing a judgement from 1965, Fuad noted that unless the accused required protection '"against himself"' through a Probation Order, '"perhaps the modern approach"' was to handle the issue outside of the courts entirely.[106]

Running alongside NAMH activities was a television programme, 'The Sick Mind', which consisted of a fortnightly forty-five-minute discussion between a psychiatrist—usually Bosa, German or Wood—and a chairperson. These programmes, it was hoped, would disseminate 'basic knowledge about mental health to the lay public' and so reduce stigma.[107] The show may have been modelled on a BBC series of five television programmes, broadcast in the UK in January 1957 under the title 'The Hurt Mind'. Yet while the BBC version included clips of psychiatrists interviewing patients about their experiences and staged demonstrations of electroconvulsive therapy and drug abreaction,[108] no patients appeared on the Uganda programme.[109] The popularity of the show, which was significant enough to keep the show on Uganda Television for five years, relied primarily on the personalities of those involved and the information presented by the psychiatrists. Topics reflected clinical diagnoses seen frequently at Butabika Hospital and Mulago Hospital Mental Health Clinic, including affective psychoses, schizophrenia, epilepsy, dementia and neurosyphilis. These topics, according to Wood, were surprisingly popular: 'following the episode discussing GPI and Syphilis the clinical laboratories were burdened by a huge increase in requests for Syphilis testing'.[110] While on a tour of Africa in 1968, George Burden, Secretary General of the International Bureau for Epilepsy, also participated in a discussion programme with Bosa.[111] The use of this medium was pioneering—not only were specialists working in maternal and public health, traditionally the most innovative in health education campaigns, only just starting to experiment with television, but the Ministry of Health themselves complained in 1968–1969 that while television was 'fully open to us to use....We had neither actors nor films for showing'.[112]

'The Sick Mind' attempted to humanise psychiatry, making visible the psychiatrists who had previously been restricted to the mental hospital. While most Africans were unable to afford a television set, the Uganda

Government, under Milton Obote, had pressed for the installation of large television screens in community centres across the country. While Obote's efforts were most likely prompted by political considerations, it had the effect of bringing educational programmes like 'The Sick Mind' to communities across Uganda. Certainly, German reported having the experience, 'on up-country clinic visits', of meeting patients and families who recognised him and his colleagues from his on-screen activities.[113] Yet the 'public' they were trying to reach was still limited. Indeed, while at first Burden 'felt we were to be congratulated' on the programme made with Bosa, this fell away when he learned 'that not more than 2% of the population have a T.V. set and that we would have been wiser to have asked for a radio programme'.[114] Indeed, it may have been such activities that Orley had in mind when he stressed that 'The job of mental health education is always hard. For every one success story told there may be several failures evident to all; added to which there are always plenty of lurid myths and rumours to dispel'.[115]

Whether or not 'The Sick Mind' succeeded in bringing a human face to psychiatry, it certainly politicised it. Shortly after Amin's takeover on 25 January 1971, the programme was moved to a new slot in a weekly production entitled 'Uganda Today', a weekly programme organised by Major Bob Astles, who later became notorious as 'the white rat of Uganda'.[116] The incorporation of this show may have been intended 'to show the Amin regime in a favourable light'.[117] Amin himself was among the programme's viewers, having watched the show from The Uganda Club prior to his takeover. As German recalled: 'Apparently he liked it - and one evening, having been presented with a new Polaroid camera, he photographed me on the screen and sent me the photograph'.[118] The photograph, which shows German mid-conversation, appears at first glance to be innocuous, but it could be read as an attempt at the kind of intimidation Amin became notorious for; as a sign that German, and by extension all of Uganda's psychiatrists, had come to the attention of Amin, and into a new political climate.[119]

PATIENTS

Psychiatrists and those attached to the NAMH placed themselves firmly on the side of patients, extending ideas about mental health they believed would benefit the mentally ill and their families. They did not, however, give the patients themselves a voice. Nor was there any room for traditional medicine or healers. Indeed, both Ugandan and expatriate psychiatrists were openly ambivalent on the topic of traditional medicine: while most acknowledged that traditional healers could serve a useful function in remote areas, particularly with regard to psychoneuroses, they were concerned that traditional healers might cause real harm to their patients, and so had no place in 'modern' psychiatry. Joseph Muhangi later described the skill with which a wealthy and famous traditional healer had treated patients at Kasangati, near Kampala. This healer held sessions of 30–45 minutes, during which he saw a white female figure with whom he spoke in tongues. Having witnessed this, 'hysterical patients with paralysed limbs, women who were infertile because of psychological problems, and men with impotence of psychological origin...were subsequently able to use their limbs, have babies and recover their potency respectively'.[120] Yet while Muhangi admitted that he was impressed by this, he also stressed that the healer was most likely epileptic, his technique merely 'psychodrama'. Bosa, too, questioned how some people could, on a Sunday morning, go to church, and in the evening visit a traditional healer, and certainly did not consider himself to be one of them. While he was open to the idea that his patients might derive benefits from visiting a traditional healer, he could never openly acknowledge it, lest he be seen to be practising or believing in traditional medicine.[121]

Bosa, like many other African doctors trained in the 1940s and 1950s, had been obliged to fight long and hard for recognition of his professional status, and setting himself apart as 'scientific' and 'modern' had been a vital part.[122] Yet they could not have been ignorant of the fact that for most of their patients, traditional healers were their first and preferred choice in times of distress. Indeed, patients were frequently vocal during consultations with psychiatrists about the causes of their problems, and the methods of treatment that were appropriate. One 23-year-old Ismaili man, for example, had been referred to a psychiatric ward of a general hospital following a period in which he 'had been behaving oddly, waving his hands about and beating his wife'.[123] He told the psychiatrist that he felt himself being pulled by a long figure in a red cloth, and this was causing him to become frightened and violent. On one occasion, the patient explained, the man in the red cloth took him to a cemetery and made the dead come alive, saying: 'I will make you like this. I will put you in a grave and bury you there'.[124] Certain that he had been bewitched, he told the psychiatrist that psychiatric medication would be useless, including electroconvulsive therapy. Instead, he would seek treatment from a young Ismaili woman, who would capture the spirit, reduce its size and burn it. The patient's role would be to pray and to attend the mosque for forty days.[125]

The distinction between 'modern' and 'anti-modern' practices in psychiatry was not one that was limited to the African context, but it took on particular significance given the scale of the cultural and political gulf between psychiatrists and their patients. Instead of seeking to use traditional healers as potential psychiatric 'allies' in a context where personnel was thin on the ground, it was made clear that a patient at Butabika might only be granted a period of leave to return home to consult a traditional healer with the permission of a psychiatrist.[126] It is questionable how frequently patients were allowed to do this, however, and there is evidence to suggest that some psychiatrists were not averse to attempting to alter 'traditional' beliefs they felt might be dangerous to the mental health of their patients. Orley, for example, was keen to promote the value of local understandings of mental illness in Buganda not only to assist in diagnosis, but also to suggest to patients alternative ways of looking at their own mental health. 'If one has some idea of the beliefs about an illness', Orley wrote in 1970, 'it is possible at times to modify them somewhat and to create new beliefs that may be more beneficial to the patient'.[127] *Akawango*, for instance, comprising a persistent headache, was of concern to patients because it indicated a potential 'spoiling' of the brain, 'and the anxiety resulting from such a belief can make things even worse'. As the name was derived from the word *ekiwanga*, however, meaning 'the skull', it would be possible for practitioners to explain, while giving medication, that the illness was limited to the bone, rather than the brain.[128] While Orley believed this was in the best interests of his patients, it nevertheless had ethical implications. 'A more dubious procedure', Orley continued, 'which I have used successfully in cases of epilepsy, is to tell the relatives of a patient that the tablets prevent the illness spreading to others, and so the patient need no longer be isolated. When it is seen that the tablets do in fact prevent fits as forecast, then the assumption is that the statement about the illness being no longer infectious is also true'.[129] This, Orley noted, was justified because it might help reduce the number of patients being subjected to 'enforced isolation' within communities.[130]

While traditional healers and ideas about mental illness were not given any formal place at Butabika, assumptions about the importance of 'community' in the treatment of mental illness nevertheless started to inform rehabilitation activities. Rhythm and drumming were encouraged among patients.[131] Group psychotherapy was also introduced among selected patients in 1968. On the one hand, this was premised on the desire to draw on the 'therapeutic potential' of less qualified hospital staff, such as nurses and ward sisters, to ensure that treatment went beyond solely physical therapies;[132] on the other, it was argued elsewhere in Africa that using groups brought psychiatry closer to the traditional 'social fabric' of African life.[133] The groups were unorthodox in the sense that 'gaining insight' was not emphasised, but they provided a forum in which patients could discuss how a ward could deal with a particularly disruptive patient, how patients would be greeted on their return home, and comparisons of 'European' and 'African' treatment.[134] In this, the role of the hospital staff, as Ugandans, was deemed to be key. As Wood explained, while they had no formal knowledge of 'psychology as a science...they live in a community and have experience of human relationships', they speak the same languages as the patients and 'are surprisingly interested in the patients' welfare', spending the most time with them on the wards. As with medical assistants, they were deemed to be particularly valuable to psychiatry because they were regarded as occupying a social and cultural space that was much closer to their patients than the psychiatrists.

Many of the reforms put in place at Butabika Hospital in the late 1960s and early 1970s aimed to extend the power of psychiatry through the staff who oversaw the day-to-day running of the hospital. Yet this did not render patients powerless within the institution. Many demonstrated their importance and independence by complaining about the quality of the food, expressing scepticism about the value of being required to talk constantly about their lives and anxieties, and negotiating medication and trips into Kampala to conduct small business deals.[135] Nakuzabasajja, for example, a 42-year-old cultivator and businessman from a small town beyond Kampala, frequently declared that he was being treated as a prisoner and rejected medication (saying there were too many tablets), as well as food, unless it was brought by his family from home.[136] When, after a stay of ten weeks, he was discharged from Butabika Hospital, he continued to resent what he regarded as unwanted attention from psychiatry. During a visit from a PSW, he became angry, stating that, as 'a government employee', the social worker had no business 'in my family affairs'.[137] After a few weeks, Nakuzabasajja wrote to the hospital, describing his suffering while in hospital, and making it clear that he would not return or take any more medication. Instead, he would remain at home, concentrating on his business, and seek assistance from traditional healers.[138] What such cases suggest is that when patients did co-operate, or build relationships with hospital staff, they had their own motivations for doing so.

CONCLUSION

Medical practitioners have described the years immediately leading up to Amin's expulsion of the Asian population in 1972 as something of a 'golden age' for psychiatry in Uganda. Writing in 1985, Bennett described Uganda as 'one of the countries in Africa with the most effective and innovative programmes for control of mental illness'.[139] He listed research that had been undertaken into the epidemiology of maternal mental illness, child psychiatry and the mental health problems of university students. He also highlighted training programmes in psychiatry and psychology available for medical students and psychiatric nurses.[140] Looking beyond the university, Orley claimed in 1970 that Butabika Hospital 'is now regarded as the natural replacement for the stocks of old. It is rare in these days to see patients shackled, although they are often tied with rope'.[141] Such was the importance of the institution, Orley asserted, that 'the immediate reaction to anyone who shows signs of what is thought to be unreasonable violence is to try to get them to Butabika Hospital, and while there is any sign that this behaviour might recur, the family are extremely reluctant to take the patient back home'.[142]

Certainly, the late 1960s and early 1970s saw a brief period of intense activity in psychiatry, characterised by attempts to extend the reach of mental health care through the training of auxiliaries, as well as educational activities aimed at the wider, if still limited, Ugandan public. In doing so, psychiatrists went well beyond their custodial and curative roles. Their actions were premised on a belief that psychiatry and psychiatric expertise could assist in improving mental health and well-being, as well as a conviction that psychiatrists could contribute their expertise to issues of social planning and national development. In turn, this culture of experimentation was not only made possible by a period of relative calm in Uganda's history, but a new sociopolitical context that encouraged innovation. Psychiatry responded and tried to contribute to the aims of the developmentalist state not only through interest in education and urbanisation, but by putting manpower needs at the centre of calls for reform. As Obote stressed in his Foreword to the *First Five-Year Development Plan*, the government's strategy 'will not work unless the people grasp the opportunity offered and participate wholeheartedly in this great task of economic and social development of the country. In the first and last analysis, the country's development is dependent on the people themselves'.[143] While psychiatrists remained subordinate to government officials, who in turn had their own concerns and priorities—not least finances, hierarchy and the maintenance of political control—the 1960s and early 1970s signalled an attempt to refigure the relationship between psychiatry and the Ugandan people, as well as the broader place of psychiatry within the nation. The mental hospital may have continued to represent the centre of psychiatric practice, and the only real institution available to the state for dealing with individuals certified as insane, but psychiatry now looked to mobilise other professionals in support of mental health care. While psychiatry had long relied on other professionals, notably the police and the judiciary, psychiatrists now sought to change ideas and practices, and to use them to extend the reach of psychiatry.

For all the rhetoric of change and success, there remained a large gap between intentions and 'on the ground' practices. The processes of admission, diagnosis and treatment remained haphazard and continued to follow the same patterns as they had under colonial rule. Until well into the 1970s at least, violence and proximity to the mental hospital remained the most common reasons for admission. Patients, too, continued to make decisions about their own lives and the types of treatment they believed were appropriate. Even among the new generation of psychiatric auxiliaries, the ability of psychiatrists to change ideas may have been limited. In a study examining the effect of psychiatric education on attitudes to illness among the Ganda, Orley and J. P. Leff, a psychiatrist based at the Medical Research Council, London, found that while educated urban Ugandans still held onto Ganda conceptions of mental illness as 'strong', coming from witchcraft or the actions of spirits, and not treatable through Western medicine, 'by the end of a course of psychiatric nursing these traditional constructs have virtually been abandoned'.[144] 'The most likely interpretation', however, was that 'the small group of people who opt for psychiatric nursing are highly self-selected and are already less traditional in their attitude to illness than the rest of the population'. As a result, they concluded, it was likely that 'the effect of medical education in changing traditional attitudes to illness may well appear disappointingly small'.[145]

While the effects of the psychiatric reforms of the late 1960s and early 1970s may have been limited within Uganda, the sense of shared challenges among psychiatrists in rapidly decolonising countries proved a unifying force across borders. Increasingly through the 1960s, Uganda's psychiatrists shared their approaches in journals such as *Psychopathologie Africaine*, and took part in transnational and international exchanges that aimed at developing ideas and practices on mental health care in the light of the contextually specific needs of newly independent African countries. During the 1968–1969 academic year, for example, visitors to the Department of Psychiatry included J. C. Likimani (Director of Mental Services, Kenya), A. Boroffka (Nigeria), R. Giel (Ethiopia), A. Howarth (Zambia), T. Baasher (Sudan), C. R. Swift (Tanzania) and C. C. Adomakoh (Ghana).[146] In the years following the establishment of Medical Faculties at the University of East Africa Colleges in Kenya and Tanzania, psychiatrists attached to Makerere also offered advice and expertise on curriculum development and became involved in the search for professorial heads and visiting lectureships.[147] At such meetings, the question of how best to organise mental health services in developing countries would come to dominate discussions, eventually being taken up as a key WHO concern.

NOTES

1. G. A. German, 'The Psychiatry of Poverty', *Psychopathologie Africaine* 7(1) (1971), p. 113.
2. Ibid.
3. M. M. Heaton, *Black Skin, White Coats: Nigerian Psychiatrists, Decolonization, and the Globalization of Psychiatry* (Ohio, 2013).
4. M. I. Assael et al., 'Psychiatric Disturbances During Pregnancy in a Rural Group of African Women', *Social Science & Medicine* 6(3) (1972), p. 394. On Kasangati Health Centre, see F. J. Bennett, G. A. Saxton, and A. Mugalula-Mukiibi, 'Kasangati—The Background to a Health Centre', in F. J. Bennett, ed., *Nkanga: Special Edition on Medicine and Social Sciences in East and West Africa* (Kampala, 1973).
5. J. L. Cox, 'Psychiatric Morbidity and Childbirth: A Prospective Study from Kasangati Health Centre, Kampala', *Proceedings of the Royal Society of Medicine* 69(3) (1976), pp. 221–222.

6. H. G. Egdell and J. P. Stanfield, 'Paediatric Neurology in Africa: A Ugandan Report', *British Medical Journal* (February 1972), pp. 548–552.

7. G. A. German, 'Aspects of Clinical Psychiatry in Sub-Saharan Africa', *The British Journal of Psychiatry* 121(564) (1972), pp. 461–479; C. A. Leon, 'Psychiatry in Latin America', *The British Journal of Psychiatry* 121(561) (1972), pp. 121–236; J. S. Neki, 'Psychiatry in South-East Asia', *The British Journal of Psychiatry* 123(574) (1973), pp. 257–269.

8. German, 'Aspects of Clinical Psychiatry', p. 477.

9. Ibid.

10. G. M. Carstairs, 'Psychiatric Problems of Developing Countries', *The British Journal of Psychiatry* 123(574) (1973), p. 272.

11. J. Hall, 'Some Aspects of Economic Development in Uganda', *African Affairs* 51(203) (1952), pp. 124–134; R. Reid, *A History of Modern Uganda* (Cambridge, 2017), p. 234.

12. A. B. K. Kasozi, *The Social Origins of Violence in Uganda, 1964–1985* (Montreal, 1994), p. 47.

13. A. Burton and M. Jennings, 'Introduction: The Emperor's New Clothes? Continuities in Governance in Late Colonial and Early Postcolonial East Africa', *International Journal of African Historical Studies* 40(1) (2007), pp. 13–14.

14. Uganda Government, *The First Five-Year Development Plan* (Entebbe, 1962), pp. 42, 44.

15. D. M. Anderson and R. Rathbone, 'Urban Africa: Histories in the Making', in D. M. Anderson and R. Rathbone, eds., *Africa's Urban Past* (Oxford, 2000).

16. *Mental Health Services in the Developing World: Reports on Workshops on Mental Health, Edinburgh (1968) and Kampala (1969)*, Commonwealth Foundation Occasional Paper, IV (Hove, 1969), p. 31.

17. *Mental Health Services in the Developing World*, p. 32.

18. C. Sicherman, *Becoming an African University: Makerere, 1922–2000* (Trenton, 2005), p. 153.

19. Reid, *A History of Modern Uganda*, p. 253.

20. J. C. Ssekamwa, *History and Development of Education in Uganda* (Kampala, 2000), Ch. 12.

21. A. Burton, 'The Haven of Peace Purged: Tackling the Undesirable and Unproductive Poor in Dar es Salaam, *ca.*1950s–1980s', *International Journal of African Historical Studies* 40(1) (2007), pp. 119–151.

22. F. J. Bennett, 'The Mental Health of African Students in Africa' (Unpublished Paper, 1967), as summarised in G. A. German and O. P. Arya, 'Psychiatric Morbidity Amongst a Uganda Student Population', *The British Journal of Psychiatry* 115 (1969), pp. 1323–1329.

23. German and Arya, 'Psychiatric Morbidity', p. 1323.

24. Ibid., p. 1324.
25. O. P. Arya and F. J. Bennett, 'Venereal Disease in an Elite Group (University Students) in East Africa', *British Journal of Venereal Diseases* 43 (1967), pp. 275–279.
26. German and Arya, 'Psychiatric Morbidity', p. 1328.
27. R. Prince, 'The "Brain Fag" Syndrome in Nigerian Students', *Journal of Mental Science* 106 (1960), p. 559.
28. German and Arya, 'Psychiatric Morbidity', p. 1327. See also, G. A. German and M. I. Assael, 'Achievement Stress and Psychiatric Disorders Amongst Students in Uganda', *Israel Annals of Psychiatry and Related Disciplines* 9(1) (1971), p. 33.
29. F. J. Bennett and A. Mugalula-Mukiibi, 'An Analysis of People Living Alone in a Rural Community in East Africa', *Social Science & Medicine* 1 (1967), pp. 97–115.
30. Uganda Government, *The First Five-Year Development Plan*, p. 2.
31. F. J. Bennett and M. I. Assael, 'The Mental Health of Immigrants and Refugees from Rwanda at Kasangati, Uganda', *Psychopathologie Africaine* 6(3) (1970), p. 322. See also, K. Long, 'Rwanda's First Refugees: Tutsi Exile and International Response 1959–64', *Journal of Eastern African Studies* 6(2) (2012), pp. 211–229.
32. Bennett and Assael, 'The Mental Health of Immigrants', p. 327.
33. Ibid., p. 326.
34. Ibid., p. 332.
35. A. M. Mazrui, *Political Values and the Educated Class in Africa* (Berkeley and Los Angeles, 1978), p. 254.
36. C. Sicherman, 'Ngugi's Colonial Education: "The Subversion...of the African Mind"', *African Studies Review* 38(3) (1995), pp. 11–41.
37. B. Lindfors, ed., *Africa Talks Back: Interviews with Anglophone African Authors* (Trenton, NJ, 2002), p. 197.
38. R. Bridges and M. Posnansky, 'African History at Makerere in the 1960s: A Further Perspective', *History in Africa* 31 (2004), pp. 479–482; C. Sicherman, *Becoming an African University*.
39. J. Nagenda, 'And This, At Last', in D. Cook, ed., *Origin East Africa: A Makerere Anthology* (London, 1965), p. 26.
40. J. Kariara, 'The Dream of Africa', in Cook, ed., *Origin East Africa*, p. 100.
41. Bennett and Assael, 'The Mental Health of Immigrants'; Bennett and Mugalula-Mukiibi, 'An Analysis of People Living Alone'.
42. Arya and Bennett, 'Venereal Disease in an Elite Group'.
43. German and Arya, 'Psychiatric Morbidity'.
44. D. W. Dunlop, 'Health Care Financing: Recent Experience in Africa', Conference paper delivered at 'Health and Development in Africa', University of Bayreuth, Germany, 2–4 June 1982, p. 13.

45. Uganda Ministry of Health Archives (UMOHA) (First and Second Five-Year Development Plans—1961/66 and 1966/71), 'Achievements', 23 April 1968, p. 1.

46. As cited in J. Iliffe, *East African Doctors: A History of the Modern Profession* (Kampala, 2002), p. 137.

47. UMOHA, PH/ASC/42, Box 56, Old Arrangement (Mental Health Advisory Committee: Association), f. 1, 'Recommendations of the Mental Health Advisory Committee on Up-Country Psychiatric Units', October 1967, p. 3

48. Ibid., p. 1.

49. Personal communication with G. A. German, 29 January 2012.

50. UMOHA PH/ASC/42, f. 6, 'Minutes of the Mental Health Advisory Committee Meeting held on 11 August 1971 in Mulago Hospital Board Room at 2.15 p.m.'.

51. UMOHA PH/ASC/42, E. B. Ssekabembe, 'Report on the Mental Health Follow Up Clinic at Jinja by Dr. Ssekabembe', n.d.; UMOHA PH/ASC/42, S. B. Bosa and F. J. Harris, 'Memorandum on the Function, Training & Recruitment of Psychiatric Social Workers & Mental Health Assistants in Uganda', no date; and UMOHA PH/ASC/42, H. G. Egdell, 'Interpreters & the Uganda Psychiatric Service', 7 October 1968.

52. UMOHA PH/ASC/42, f. 3, 'Minutes of the 11th Meeting of the Mental Health Advisory Committee held on 24 June 1969', p. 1.

53. UMOHA PH/ASC/42, Egdell, 'Interpreters', 7 October 1968.

54. Ibid.

55. UMOHA PH/ASC/42, f. 3, 'Minutes of the 11th Meeting of the Mental Health Advisory Committee held on 24 June 1969', p. 1.

56. UMOHA PH/ASC/42, 'Memorandum on the Function, Training & Recruitment of Psychiatric Social Workers & Mental Health Assistants in Uganda'.

57. UMOHA PH/ASC/42, f. 2, 'Minutes of the 9th Meeting of the Mental Health Advisory Committee held on 29 October 1968', p. 2.

58. UMOHA PH/ASC/42, 'Report on the Mental Health Follow Up Clinic at Jinja by Dr. Ssekabembe', p. 1.

59. UMOHA PH/ASC/42, S. Beyo Bosa, 'Report on the Development and Functioning of the Psychiatric Clinic at Mbarara Hospital, Ankole District', n.d. (likely 1969), p. 2.

60. Ibid., p. 3.

61. Personal communication with German.

62. UMOHA C90/ACR (Bosa Stephen B—Consult. Psychiat.), f. 113, letter from J. Bulwanyi, Medical Superintendent, to The Permanent Secretary/Chief Medical Officer, Entebbe, 3 April 1967.

63. J. Orley, 'A Prospective Study of 372 Consecutive Admissions to Butabika Hospital, Kampala', *East African Medical Journal* 49(1) (1972), p. 18.
64. UMOHA C90/ACR, f. 127, letter from Y. K. Lule, Principal, Makerere University College, to I. S. Kadama, Chief Medical Officer, Entebbe, 27 July 1968.
65. F. J. Bennett, 'Medical Manpower in East Africa: Prospects and Problems', *East African Medical Journal* 42(4) (1965), pp. 149–161.
66. H. G. Egdell, 'The Medical Assistant and Psychiatric Care', *Psychopathologie Africaine* 6 (1970), p. 83.
67. UMOHA PH/ASC/42, 'Memorandum on the Training of Medical Assistants in Psychiatry', 24 June 1969.
68. Egdell, 'The Medical Assistant', p. 83.
69. Ibid.
70. Ibid., p. 85.
71. UMOHA PH/ASC/42, 'Memorandum on the Training of Medical Assistants in Psychiatry', 24 June 1969.
72. UMOHA PH/ASC/42, f. 3, 'Minutes of the 11th Meeting of the Mental Health Advisory Committee Held on 24 June 1969', p. 2.
73. UMOHA PH/ASC/42, S. Beyo Bosa, 'Report on the Development and Functioning of the Psychiatric Clinic at Mbarara Hospital, Ankole District', n.d. (likely 1969), p. 3; UMOHA PH/ASC/42, 'Report on the Mental Health Follow Up Clinic at Jinja by Dr. Ssekabembe', p. 1.
74. UMOHA PH/ASC/42, 'Memorandum on the Training of Medical Assistants in Psychiatry', 24 June 1969.
75. UMOHA PH/ASC/42, f. 6, 'Minutes of the Mental Health Advisory Committee Meeting Held on 11 August 1971 in Mulago Hospital Board Room at 2.15 p.m.', p. 1.
76. Interview with female nurse (RUK-10), Rwakabengo, Rukungiri, 5 July 2011.
77. Orley, 'A Prospective Study', p. 21.
78. Ibid., p. 18.
79. J. F. Wood, 'A Half Century of Growth in Ugandan Psychiatry', *Uganda Atlas of Disease Distribution* (Kampala, 1968), p. 121.
80. 'Question 18 of 1970, 21 April 1970', *Uganda Hansard*, 99, Fourth Session (1970/1971), pp. 18–20.
81. J. F. Wood, 'An Introduction to the Uganda Psychiatric Service' (Unpublished lecture, copy in possession of author, 1969).
82. J. F. Wood, 'Psychiatry for Lawyers' (Unpublished lecture, copy in possession of author, 1970).
83. Wood, 'Psychiatry for Lawyers'.

84. Wood, 'Psychiatry for Lawyers'; Roger Davidson, 'Psychiatry and Homosexuality in Mid-Twentieth-Century Edinburgh: The View from Jordanburn Nerve Hospital', *History of Psychiatry* 20(4) (2009), p. 417.

85. B. J. F. Laubscher, *Sex, Custom and Psychopathology: A Study of South African Pagan Natives* (London, 1937); A. H. Leighton et al., eds., *Psychiatric Disorders Among the Yoruba: A Report from the Cornell-Aro Mental Health Research Project in the Western Region, Nigeria* (Ithaca, NY, 1963), p. 111; C. G. F. Smartt, 'Mental Maladjustment in the East African', *British Journal of Mental Science* 102 (1956), p. 442; W. H. Watson, 'A Case of Sexual Perversion in an African Male', *East African Medical Journal* 20(10) (1943), p. 354. On psychiatry and homosexuality in South Africa, see T. F. Jones, *Psychiatry, Mental Institutions, and the Mad in Apartheid South Africa* (Abingdon, 2012), Ch. 7.

86. German and Arya, 'Psychiatric Morbidity', pp. 1323–1329.

87. On the history of attitudes to homosexuality, see K. Cheney, 'Locating Neocolonialism, "Tradition," and Human Rights in Uganda's "Gay Death Penalty"', *African Studies Review* 55(2) (2012), pp. 77–95; N. Hoad, *African Intimacies: Race, Homosexuality, and Globalization* (Minneapolis, 2007), Ch. 1; S. Tamale, 'Out of the Closet: Unveiling Sexuality Discourses in Uganda', in C. M. Cole, T. Manuh, and S. F. Miescher, eds., *Africa After Gender* (Bloomington, IN, 2007), p. 10.

88. CAP 302, *The Penal Code Act* (Entebbe, 1950).

89. Uganda Protectorate, *Annual Report of the Judiciary for the Year Ended 31st December, 1960* (Entebbe, 1961), p. 2.

90. Wood, 'Psychiatry for Lawyers'.

91. Wood, 'Psychiatry for Lawyers'.

92. D. L. Davies, 'Report on the Teaching of Psychiatry at Makerere University College Department of Psychiatry' (Unpublished report, copy in possession of author, 1969); Personal communication with German.

93. Wood, 'An Introduction to the Uganda Psychiatric Service'.

94. Personal communication with J. F. Wood, 7 October 2011.

95. Wood, 'An Introduction to the Uganda Psychiatric Service'.

96. *Mental Health Services in the Developing World*, p. 43.

97. Personal communication with German; 'Department of Psychiatry Annual Report, 1968–1969', *Makerere University College Reports, 1968–1969* (Kampala, copy in possession of author, 1969).

98. Kenya, for example, did not start a National Mental Health Association until 1986. World Health Organization Library (WHOL) MNH/POL/87.3, *Tenth Meeting of the African Mental Health Action Group, Geneva, 8 May 1987*, p. 5.

99. Bodleian Library, University of Oxford (BOD) Micr.Afr.609(2) (Papers of J. N. P. Davies), 'Mental Hospital Annual Report, 1956', p. 5; G. I. Tewfik, 'A Hospital Visitors' Association', *The Lancet* (October 1956), p. 834.

100. UMOHA PH/ASC/42.

101. Personal communication with German.
102. A. M. Tripp, *Women and Politics in Uganda* (Oxford, 2000), Ch. 2.
103. UMOHA PH/ASC/42, 'Notes from the Chairman's Report to the A.G.M.', 5 December 1970; Personal communication with German.
104. UMOHA PH/ASC/42, 'Uganda National Association for Mental Health membership form', n.d.
105. J. Fuad, 'Insanity and the Law' (Unpublished seminar paper, copy in possession of author, 1970).
106. Fuad, 'Insanity and the Law'.
107. 'Department of Psychiatry Report, 1966–1967', *Makerere University College Reports, 1966–1967* (Kampala, copy in possession of author, 1967); Personal communication with German. On Uganda Television see Abraham Z. Bass, 'Promoting Nationhood Through Television in Africa', *Journal of Broadcasting* 13(2) (1969), p. 164; Deborah Haskell, 'Educational Television in Uganda', *Today's Speech* 19(4) (1971), pp. 43–49.
108. G. M. Carstairs and J. K. Wing, 'Attitudes of the General Public to Mental Illness', *British Medical Journal* (6 September 1958), pp. 594–597. A selection of clips from this series is available on YouTube: British Broadcasting Corporation, 'Physical Mental Health Treatments 1957, Part 1', last accessed 12 December 2012, at http://www.youtube.com/watch?v=2KxU3dPeink.
109. Personal communication with Wood.
110. Personal communication with Wood.
111. World Health Organization Archives (WHOA) M4/348/1 (General Information re: Relations with Mental Health Organisations, Jkt 1), f. 73, George Burden, 'Africa Revisited—December 1968', p. 3.
112. UMOHA GCH 9/2 (Health Education), f. 140(2), 'Plan of Work for Health Education Unit of Ministry of Health Basis for Wider Planning', 1969, p. 3; F. J. Bennett and H. Senkatuka, 'Health Education Via Mass Media', *Journal of Tropical Pediatrics* 12(supp3) (1966), pp. 31–32.
113. Personal communication with German.
114. WHOA M4/348/1, f. 73, Burden, 'Africa Revisited', p. 3.
115. Orley, *Culture and Mental Illness*, p. 57.
116. Personal communication with German; Haskell, 'Educational Television'. On Astles, see 'Obituaries: Bob Astles', *The Times*, 23 January 2013; Paul Vallely, 'I Genuinely Felt That by Being There I Could Moderate His Excesses', *The Times*, 10 December 1985, p. 5.
117. Personal communication with German.
118. Personal communication with German.
119. On Amin's use of the media see Patrick Keatley, 'Obituary: Idi Amin', *The Guardian*, 18 August 2003; D. R. Peterson and E. C. Taylor, 'Rethinking the State in Idi Amin's Uganda: The Politics of Exhortation', *Journal of Eastern African Studies* 7(1) (2013), pp. 58–82.

120. J. Muhangi, 'Psychiatry in Kenya: New Horizons in Medical Care', Inaugural lecture delivered at the University of Nairobi, 31 January 1980, pp. 15–16.
121. Personal communication with Joseph Bossa, 6 July 2012.
122. Iliffe, *East African Doctors*, Ch. 5. Much of this fight can be traced through UMOHA PH/ASC/46 (Box 29) (Makerere Medical Graduates Association).
123. F. J. Harris, *Social Casework: An Introduction for Students in Developing Countries* (Nairobi, 1970), p. 161.
124. Ibid.
125. Ibid., pp. 160–165.
126. Personal communication with German; Personal communication with Wood.
127. Orley, *Culture and Mental Illness*, p. 52.
128. Ibid.
129. Ibid., p. 53.
130. Ibid.
131. Personal communication with Wood.
132. J. F. Wood, 'Utilising Therapeutic Potential in Psychiatric Hospital Staff', *Psychopathologie Africaine* 6(3) (1970), p. 301. The importance of small social groups is also emphasised in J. F. Wood, 'Rehabilitation & Psychiatry' (Unpublished lecture, copy in possession of author, n.d.).
133. E. Corin and H. B. M. Murphy, 'Psychiatric Perspectives in Africa Part I: The Western Viewpoint', *Transcultural Psychiatry* 16(2) (1979), p. 168; T. A. Lambo, 'Psychotherapy in Africa', *Psychotherapy and Psychosomatics* 24(4–6) (1974), pp. 311–326.
134. Lambo, 'Psychotherapy in Africa', pp. 312, 314.
135. Harris, *Social Casework*.
136. Ibid., pp. 142–149.
137. Ibid., p. 148.
138. Ibid., p. 146.
139. F. J. Bennett, as cited in C. P. Dodge and P. D. Wiebe, eds., *Crisis in Uganda: The Breakdown of Health Services* (Oxford, 1985), p. 50.
140. Ibid.
141. Orley, *Culture and Mental Illness*, p. 30.
142. Ibid., p. 41.
143. Uganda Government, *First Five Year Development Plan*, Foreword.
144. J. H. Orley and J. P. Leff, 'The Effect of Psychiatric Education on Attitudes to Illness Among the Ganda', *The British Journal of Psychiatry* 121(2) (1972), p. 140.
145. Ibid.
146. 'Department of Psychiatry Report, 1968–1969'.
147. Personal communication with German.

CHAPTER 6

Mobility, Power and International Mental Health

In 1960, seventeen newly independent countries, most of them African, became formal member states of the United Nations (UN). This number grew over the next decade, with Uganda's application ratified in 1962, so that by 1970 the decolonising world was the dominant power within the UN. This shift in the balance of power would significantly alter debates and policy formation from the 1960s, not least within the World Health Organization (WHO), which now had to contend with the demands of new member states for economic development.[1] Addressing the World Federation of Mental Health (WFMH) in 1961, Maria Pfister, Medical Officer in the Mental Health Section of the WHO, described how 'the dynamic characteristics' of the shift in membership 'is felt throughout the Organization, and the rapidly increasing number of countries gaining independence has led to a corresponding increase in the number of health programmes being planned and set up in conjunction with WHO', especially in Africa.[2] In addition to responding to requests for emergency assistance, the WHO was setting up long-term training programmes in a range of health-related subjects in developing countries, seeking new collaborative research links and broadening the membership of its Expert Advisory Committees.[3] In 1961, the Eleventh Expert Committee on Mental Health, which discussed the role of public health officers and general practitioners in mental health care, comprised eight psychiatrists from around the world, including Thomas Adeoye Lambo (Nigeria), Jose Horwitz (Chile) and W. A. Karunaratne

© The Author(s) 2019
Y. Pringle, *Psychiatry and Decolonisation in Uganda*,
Mental Health in Historical Perspective,
https://doi.org/10.1057/978-1-137-60095-0_6

(Ceylon).[4] The following year, among the seven psychiatrists attending the Twelfth Expert Committee on Mental Health, which looked at the training of psychiatrists, were Taha A. Baasher (Khartoum), Tsung-yi Lin (Taiwan) and Ignacio Matte Blanco (Chile).[5] While during the early 1960s, as Pfister herself stressed to the WFMH, the WHO made no explicit distinction between developed and developing countries in their mental health policy, this changed over the next decade. The rise of a New International Economic Order within the UN General Assembly, focused on promoting economic and social development in developing countries, found expression within the WHO in calls to address systemic disparities in health between developed and developing countries.[6]

This emergent language of global structural inequality, as well as 'developing countries' as a distinct bloc with its own challenges and needs, pervaded the Sixteenth Expert Committee on Mental Health, which considered the organisation of mental health services in developing countries. Meeting in 1974, the Committee stressed that over forty million men, women and children were suffering from 'serious untreated mental disorders' in developing countries, and that mental health could not be considered in isolation from social and economic development.[7] 'In planning services', according to Norman Sartorius, a Croatian psychiatrist and Chief Medical Officer of the WHO's Office of Mental Health, 'standards from countries in the United States and Europe are often taken as the objective to be reached, although both planners and psychiatrists fully realize the impossibility of reaching it; what is worse is that even if these objectives should be achieved, it is questionable whether they would lead to optimal service delivery patterns'.[8] In line with the new political climate, it was increasingly argued that developing countries needed to define their own needs and objectives, taking into account what was possible in the short term in poor socio-economic settings. This context-specific approach to policy marked a departure from the WHO's more usual technocratic approach, in which the systematic collection and comparison of information was used to define universal norms and standards. While psychiatrists in countries around the world had increasingly experimented with mental health care and the extension of psychiatry beyond institutions since the late 1950s, by 1974 the WHO had not yet attempted methodologically rigorous research on the organisation and effectiveness of these new approaches. Despite this, the WHO sought to provide strategic guidance on how psychiatry and mental health care in developing countries might best be developed. The *Report* of the Expert Committee, published in 1975, recommended that member states in developing countries should move to decentralise mental health services, integrate mental health care with general health services, and allow for the sharing of mental health tasks between psychiatrists, a wide range of health workers, and community agencies.[9] This broadly-conceived version of mental health in primary care would become the major plank of WHO policy on mental health over the next three decades.

This chapter explores the ways that psychiatrists—particularly African psychiatrists—mobilised and shared ideas on strategies for improving mental health care from the early 1960s. It does so in order to trace the roots of the WHO's policy of mental health in primary care. Uganda was one of a range of countries whose model of training and delegating responsibility to a range of health care workers attracted the interest of staff attached to the WHO's Office of Mental Health. Temporally, this chapter overlaps with the reforms within Uganda discussed in Chapter 5, but instead explores how ideas about the organisation of mental health care, and what this might mean for the future of psychiatry as a profession, were discussed in an increasingly focused manner at regional and international meetings through the 1960s. The psychiatrists explored in Chapter 5 never intended their activities to remain limited to the local or national context, but sought to inform a more contextually sensitive psychiatry elsewhere. The discussions held among psychiatrists from across Africa highlight the variety of models still being explored in national contexts by the early 1970s, disagreements about the extent to which psychiatry could be delegated to others and shared concerns about the social and cultural gulf between psychiatrists and their patients. At the same time, they also raise questions about mobility and the power of psychiatrists, either individually, or as a group of 'African psychiatrists' or psychiatrists from 'developing countries'. And they can help us understand why some countries (or indeed individual psychiatrists) were more dominant than others. The capacity of psychiatrists to contribute both to an increasingly transnational and global body of ideas about mental health care was shaped by a wide range of factors, not least political stability, the availability of funding, and sufficient manpower within their own countries to allow psychiatrists to travel and participate in international mental health. This was no less the case in Uganda as it was elsewhere. The opening of the Department of Psychiatry in 1966 not only increased the number of psychiatrists able to experiment with mental health care, but allowed professional freedom and the financial means (if still limited) to travel, particularly among those whose contracts included research. The political and economic turmoil that followed Idi Amin's takeover of the country in January 1971, however, and the conflict and violence that continued into the 1980s, saw most of the expatriate psychiatrists leave the country, and Ugandan psychiatrists flee into exile. After 1973, Uganda's role in international mental health was limited to those psychiatrists now in the diaspora.

The Making of an 'African' Psychiatric Tradition

The professionalisation of psychiatry in Africa coincided with decolonisation and increased interest in the mental health problems of the rapidly decolonising world within international mental health. In this context, it was politically important to many of those attending the first international meetings on psychiatry and mental illness in Africa to push back against the biodeterminism that had been espoused by ethnopsychiatry and to demonstrate the universality of the human psyche. The first major 'Meeting of Specialists on Mental Health' in Africa, held in Bukavu in March 1958 under the auspices of the Commission for Technical Co-operation in Africa South of the Sahara (CCTA), the WFMH and the WHO, concluded that psychiatrists should aspire to global uniformity in their ideas about and responses to mental illness. While attention should be given to 'the particular ethnic, cultural and social conditions prevailing in this continent', the final report noted, psychiatric approaches should be broadly the same as in other continents.[10] Notions of equality and unity were also at the forefront of the First Pan-African Psychiatric Conference, organised by Thomas A. Lambo in Nigeria in November 1961, just one year after Nigerian Independence. In using the conference to emphasise the 'unity of mankind', Lambo, to borrow a phrase from Matthew Heaton, was attempting 'to insert cultural politics into a psychiatric framework'.[11]

The politically conscious nature of these early meetings of psychiatrists made many feel uneasy about the unequal distribution of the participants. Of the thirty-four delegates attending the meeting in Bukavu, only twelve were psychiatric professionals practising in Africa and, with the exceptions of Tigani el Mahi (Sudan), E. B. Forster (Ghana), A. C. Raman (Mauritius) and Abraham Ordia (Nigeria), all were expatriates. G. I. Tewfik attended as representative for Uganda, and had to confess to the group that he had 'so little personal experience' that he could only review the literature on psychosis in Africa, drawing heavily on J. C. Carothers' monograph *The African Mind in Health and Disease*, rather than presenting a context-specific analysis of Uganda.[12] Three years later, in Nigeria, Lambo attempted to rectify the situation somewhat, bringing together ninety-two participants from twenty-two countries in Africa, Europe and the USA. These included major figures in transcultural psychiatry, such as Alexander H. Leighton and Sir Aubrey Lewis, the founder of the WFMH, John R. Rees, and E. E. Krapf, Chief Medical Officer of Mental Health at the WHO. Forster and El-Mahi were also in attendance, as well as T. W. Murray, as representative for Uganda.[13] Yet psychiatrists working in Africa were again outnumbered at the conference, leading to frustration, among some, that international delegates were 'Inexperienced in the sense that their view of African problems was rarely based on the reality of the African situation, and tended to be heavily influenced by theoretical formulations and current Western attitudes and ideologies concerning developing countries and "primitive" societies'.[14]

At the end of the First Pan-African Psychiatric Conference, Lambo called for the creation of a professional association 'meant entirely for psychiatrists working in Africa; actively engaged in some form of mental health work in Africa, irrespective of their origin or nationalities'.[15] In order to be in a position to ensure that discussion of mental illness in Africa was focused on practical realities, psychiatrists needed to engage in close collaboration with colleagues from across the continent. The proposal represented a call to decolonise psychiatric practices as well as an appeal to a sense of common challenges facing psychiatrists working in Africa. This included professional isolation (both from other branches of medicine and from other psychiatrists), ongoing underdevelopment and neglect by national governments, and the social and cultural gap between psychiatrists and their patients—a gap that had not been resolved through Africanisation. It was this sense of shared experience, more than any appeal to African unity, that provided a common starting point for psychiatrists in Africa, and which required an inclusive approach to membership.

Despite agreement as to the need for a professional body of psychiatrists in Africa, the establishment of an association proved impractical in 1961 due to the size of the continent and a lack of funds for regular meetings. While international organisations like the WHO and the

WFMH were increasingly making small sums available to assist with conference organisation, attendance and training, a long-term commitment for an association was not forthcoming. Instead, eight psychiatrists, including Lambo, Tolani Asuni (Nigeria), Henri Collomb (Senegal) and Raman, agreed to create 'a feeling of association' through correspondence and an agreement to organise a conference every five years. Overall, the correspondence system was not a success, with workloads preventing regular correspondence between most.[16] One exception appears to have been between G. Allen German, of Makerere University College, Uganda, and Asuni, whose brief visit to Uganda in 1967 was unexpectedly extended by a short period when the outbreak of the Nigerian-Biafran war prevented his return home. According to German, a warm friendship was sparked between the two and, having discovered common psychiatric viewpoints, an active correspondence ensued.[17]

The situation was different when the idea of an association was again raised in the late 1960s: not only had the number of psychiatrists in Africa increased significantly (in relative terms, at least), but international organisations were investing more in mental health. Following further discussions at the Second Pan-African Psychiatric Conference in Dakar, Senegal, in 1968, the Association of Psychiatrists in Africa was eventually launched at the workshop on 'Mental Health Services in Developing Countries' in Kampala in April 1969, with Asuni elected as its first President. The workshop was recognised as a fitting venue for the official launch of the Association because it was the first meeting on the continent at which psychiatrists working in Africa were in the majority. Generous funding from the Commonwealth Foundation meant that twenty-two of the twenty-nine delegates were from Africa, with representatives from Ghana, Kenya, Nigeria, Sudan, Ethiopia, Zambia, Tanzania and Mauritius. Seven psychiatrists in Uganda, including Stephen B. Bosa, unable to attend other meetings due to a flying phobia, were also in attendance.[18] The composition therefore fit with the Association's aim of taking 'the lead in promoting developments in psychiatry within Africa and in speaking to the outside world with a relatively united voice'.[19] While all were broadly in agreement that transcultural psychiatric research had so far demonstrated the universality of mental illness and the human psyche, there remained debate over the future of psychiatry in Africa, and the extent to which social, cultural and economic circumstances demanded that psychiatry be different to that elsewhere.

The discussion at the workshop highlighted a wide variety of experiments in new ways of providing mental health care already underway. These included village settlements in Tanzania and Nigeria, which raised concerns among delegates about cost, staffing and stigma.[20] Baasher offered a 'striking example' of his own practice in Sudan, where he described rejecting the mental hospital 'on the grounds of distance and divorce from local culture'.[21] Instead, he had asked for beds in district hospitals, drawing on the additional support of traditional healers and prison authorities in what could be termed 'a spread-out mental hospital'.[22] H. G. Egdell described the development of new psychiatric units in remote rural hospitals in Uganda, staffed by a new grade of medical assistant who was 'the key one in the development of rural psychiatric services'.[23] Several others, meanwhile, remained enthusiastic about the ongoing importance of large mental hospitals, emphasising their complexity and 'necessity for good record keeping'.[24] Yet while all were dealing with similar legacies stemming from colonial rule, there was no clear consensus on how mental health care might be best reorganised. There was broad agreement about the need for more support for psychiatrists, in some form or another, deemed essential to extending the reach of psychiatry given the lack of specialist personnel and limited resources. Yet the definition, training, and responsibility of these additional workers remained a matter of contention. While Charles R. Swift, psychiatrist in Tanzania, defined the auxiliary as 'someone who helps a member of the psychiatric team', Egdell pushed for a more specialist understanding, with responsibilities to assist general medical officers, assist the psychiatrist and 'trained to take on a certain amount of responsibility to provide continuity of care, and even leadership in times of crisis'.[25] Stressing the linguistic and cultural problems of understanding patients, Mrs. A. P. White, a sociologist and research assistant with the Department of Psychiatry, suggested the development of a new grade of auxiliary, 'the patient's friend', someone with only very basic training in psychiatry, 'to whom the patient would be assigned following his initial contact with the doctor and who would act as an intermediary'.[26] Meanwhile, J. W. S. Kasirye, Medical Superintendent of Butabika Hospital, added that he believed there was scope for health visitors to be used as 'case "spotters"', but he did not think that they, 'as medical assistants, could undertake a therapeutic role'.[27]

Underlying these disagreements were concerns both about the ability of auxiliaries to care for patients with major mental illness and justifiable fears about psychiatrists' hard-won, but still insecure professional status within their home countries. Changes in the organisation and delivery of mental health care had implications for the nature of psychiatric practice, with more time spent supervising and training health workers, social workers and other related professionals. Such concerns over status were not limited to psychiatrists in Africa. In debates on mental health care in Asia, too, were concerns that while additional manpower was necessary, particularly among nurses and auxiliaries, psychiatrists needed to work to overcome any 'demarcation disputes'. As Carstairs noted on India, what psychiatrist would really want to work in a supervisory role in an up-country clinic? In a statement that recalls the use of remote postings as a punishment for dissent under colonial rule, he added: 'Young doctors all aspire to work in towns, either in large well-equipped hospitals or in lucrative private practice'.[28]

Disagreements over the use of psychiatric auxiliaries reflected broader uncertainty about the role psychiatrists should have in Africa, and the workshop and Association provided the first opportunity for collective discussion on what the role of the psychiatrist in Africa might be. On this question, some were uneasy about taking on too much responsibility beyond that which they had been trained. Adomakoh 'cautioned the psychiatrists against accepting too wide a social advisory role because of their over intense need to please'.[29] A. Boroffka, meanwhile, argued that while health promotion and the advising of educationists, economists and town planners were 'fascinating and attractive', and psychiatrists should prepare themselves for those tasks, for the time being they should be modest in their outlook. As there were so few psychiatrists in Africa, an advisory role 'borders on betrayal of our professional ethics....One also may loose [sic.] one's expertness in psychiatry if one stops seeing patients'.[30] Others at the meeting disagreed, arguing that 'the psychiatrist could not be so confined, particularly in a developing society where his intelligence and expertise are at a premium. He must be prepared to take on many mantles, and must be prepared to offer advice in those areas of social planning which were likely to influence the mental health and happiness of people'.[31] Whatever individual psychiatrists might see their roles as being, however, they were likely to come up against resistance from administrators and other leaders, their being 'slow to recognise more than a custodial and curative role for mental health experts'.[32] The question of what 'African' psychiatry should be was not resolved here, and nor did the delegates necessarily believe that it should be. Despite their common challenges, they recognised the vast differences that existed not only between countries but within them. More important, was a common sense that creativity was necessary—what Diop later explained to the African Regional Committee of the WHO as the need for flexibility in the reorganisation of existing mental health services, and for countries to 'innovate according to their circumstances and the requirements of community psychiatry'.[33] It was this need for innovation and for the involvement of psychiatric auxiliaries that WHO officials would find most appealing in debates about the future of mental health care.

THE WHO AND MENTAL HEALTH IN PRIMARY CARE

In the decades following the Second World War, the WHO, the WFMH, and the Commonwealth Foundation provided funding that enabled psychiatrists in developing countries to participate in international mental health. These most frequently took the form of small regional meetings, involving less travel, fewer costs and allowing closer dialogue between people who shared similar professional and socio-cultural conditions. They provided spaces for the sharing of ideas, the establishment of general principles and practical strategies for raising psychiatry and mental health as a priority among national planners. As Senegalese psychiatrist S. M. B. Babakar Diop stressed in 1973, 'everything may seem to have priority when it is a question of establishing a nation, uniting a country', and ensuring that everyone had access to food, education, medical care and work.[34] These meetings did not achieve, or even aim at identifying uniformity in approaches to psychiatry and mental health care, however. Just as delegates at the workshop in Kampala in 1969 highlighted the range of approaches required to account for the wide variation in geographical, social, cultural and economic conditions, so did those at a conference on the organisation of mental health services in India in 1971. Organised by the Indian Psychiatric Association and sponsored by the WFMH, the final report stressed that because of this diversity, there was not only 'an opportunity' but 'a need to experiment with different methods of delivering mental health care'.[35]

While the WHO facilitated these discussions by helping to organise meetings throughout the 1960s, it was not until the early 1970s that the WHO's Office of Mental Health, as represented by Sartorius, Harding and Joy Moser, started to outline priorities for the development of mental health services in developing countries. These included the need to establish what types of mental illness were suitable for intervention on a wide scale, what innovations in mental health care were already underway in member states, and the development of pilot programmes to test and evaluate the operation of these strategies. Above all, was a concern to promote the 'development of front-line mental health manpower to meet the needs of local areas, and collaboration with existing health services'.[36] This was in line both with the WHO's own priorities as a public health organisation and with the approaches being trialled in contexts around the world. Harding referred to the success of 'innovative efforts' to train and 'include in the care of the mentally ill those who previously had no mental health function'. He cited programmes for the training of assistants in Uganda, Zambia, and Sarawak, public health nurses in Colombia, and traditional healers and the wider community at Aro, Nigeria, under Lambo.[37] Moser similarly reported on Tanzanian medical auxiliaries who had received a week's intensive training, a programme to train Zambian psychiatric medical assistants ('mini-psychiatrists'), and schemes in Uganda to train medical assistants who could assist in district hospitals and who were 'trained to take on a certain amount of responsibility for continuity of care, and even leadership in times of crisis'.[38]

Many of the experiments in reorganising mental health care resonated with the WHO officials because they presupposed an integrated approach to public and mental health. In the context of broader calls within the UN for social and economic development in developing countries, the need for a strategy for mental health care had taken on a new urgency, and the experiences of psychiatrists in developing countries provided a body of practical examples as to how this might be achieved. Mental health was already being overlooked in the high-level intra-agency meetings between the World Health Assembly and the UNICEF/WHO Joint Committee on Health Policy (JCHP) on primary health care which would culminate in the 1978 Alma-Ata Declaration, and clear policy was needed. As Harding summarised in the opening statements to the WHO Seminar on the Organization of Mental Health Services in Addis Ababa, 1973, there was 'a need to be much more specific than in the past in defining mental health services'. Instead of 'imprecise requests for services described with a blanket reference to "mental health" or "psychiatry"', psychiatrists needed to be prepared to make their case with reference to financial implications, target populations, personnel management and potential health outcomes. So too should psychiatrists be wary of proposing too many changes at once. As

Harding cautioned, 'The risk is that this becomes a shopping list presented to the health planner whose first thought will be the enormous expense of such a "comprehensive" service. The temptation will be to provide little or nothing'.[39]

From 1973, Sartorius, Harding and Moser consulted widely with psychiatrists from around the world. With the express intention of drawing up suggestions for WHO action, Moser toured nine African countries in late 1973, attending a meeting of the Association of Psychiatrists in Africa in Lagos, Nigeria, at which the Association provided a unified position on the importance of psychiatric auxiliaries in mental health care in Africa. She also attended the WHO Africa Regional Committee, also in Nigeria, whose technical discussion was on the place of mental health in public health.[40] Harding, meanwhile, attended a seminar on the organisation of mental health services held under the auspices of the WHO's Regional Office for the Eastern Mediterranean in Addis Ababa in November-December 1973, and whose participants included Narendra N. Wig (India), Collomb, Asuni, Ravi L. Kapur (India) and A. Kamal (Iraq). Harding's attendance and introductory paper presented at the meeting was explicitly intended 'to draw together some of the key issues which face WHO (including its Expert Committee) as well as governments and individuals who are concerned with the problems of mental health in the developing countries'.[41] Sartorius, moreover, attended an Association of Psychiatrists in Africa workshop in Nairobi in September 1974, one month before the Expert Meeting on the Organisation of Mental Health Services in Developing Countries. One afternoon, German recalled, he was invited to join Sartorius and other WHO colleagues to discuss the methods used to extend the reach of psychiatry in Uganda, and the strategies employed where specialist personnel were scarce.[42] Such discussions would only have reinforced existing sentiment that the lack of psychiatrists meant that the extension of mental health services required the use of new types of personnel as well as a reorientation of the relationship between psychiatry and other institutions and services.

The Sixteenth Expert Committee on Mental Health met in Geneva in October 1974, bringing together ten expert members, including Wig, Diop, F. Workneh (Ethiopia), M. A. Bakiri (Algeria), E.-S. Tan (Malaysia) and C. A. Leon (Colombia). Taiwanese psychiatrist T.-Y. Lin was in attendance as the representative of the WFMH, and among the Secretariat were Baasher, Binitie, and Sartorius, Moser, and Harding. Over seven days, the participants discussed the extent and nature of mental health problems in developing countries, present responses, different approaches to the development of services, manpower, monitoring and evaluation, regional and international activities and drafted and finalised a final report.[43] Introduced by Lambo in his capacity as Deputy Director-General of the WHO, the *Report* stressed that the most urgent problem in the development and delivery of mental health services was adequate coverage of the population, particularly in rural areas with a widely dispersed population. The most important constraint, meanwhile, was 'the extreme scarcity of mental health professionals'—less than one per million of the population, in some countries—something that required 'fresh consideration of the role and training both of general health workers and of mental health professionals'.[44] Denouncing centralised and custodial mental hospitals as inappropriate and counter-therapeutic, the *Report* unequivocally recommended 'the decentralization of mental health services' to community, regional and district levels, the 'integration of mental health services with the general health service', and 'the development of collaboration with nonmedical community agencies' such as religious leaders, teachers and the police.[45] While some limited cooperation between health workers at the village level and traditional healers might be useful, or at least not harmful, it steered away from recommending collaboration between traditional healers and psychiatrists, and even suggested that psychiatrists might seek to exercise some form of control over their practices.[46] Cooperation with those working in general health services, instead, would be the priority. In consequence, a major part of the psychiatrists' role in developing countries would involve providing basic training for less specialist personnel, supervision for health workers and limited care for only the most difficult cases. This, according to R. Giel and Harding, was in alignment not only with shifts already underway in many developing countries, but with the redirection of WHO programmes towards the strengthening of basic health services through primary health workers.[47]

The Expert Committee had made its recommendations on the basis of a collected body of knowledge and experience from psychiatrists in developing countries over the previous decade. These had shown that with only minimal financial investment, 'improved mental health care in developing countries was not an unattainable ideal'.[48] This approach to policy formation was problematic, however, being in opposition to the

WHO's preferred technocratic method of systematic research and data collection. Within only a few months of the publication of the *Report*, concerns started to be raised that there was no evidence that primary health workers could manage major psychiatric illness, and without this they could not persuade political leaders to include it as an approach in national health policy.[49] It was evidence that could be used for standard- and policy-making that the WHO Collaborative Study on Strategies for Extending Mental Health Care took as its main objective. Starting in 1975, pilot programmes were established in seven countries—Brazil, Colombia, Egypt, India, the Philippines, Senegal and Sudan—to assess the feasibility and effectiveness of different techniques for community-based mental health care, training methods for health workers, and the roles that might be played by those not directly concerned with health, such as the police.[50] Yet even this proved unsuccessful: a lack of resources and personnel rendered any sophisticated evaluation of these programmes impossible, resulting in a lack of any useful comparable data between them. Despite this, participation in the study alone confirmed to the WHO the value of mental health in primary care. The ability of primary health workers to provide mental health care, it was observed, was serving to change attitudes towards the mentally ill among health personnel, administrators and health planners in the study areas: 'Initial resistance...soon developed into general acceptance of the use of primary health workers'.[51] This ideal of the integration and delegation of mental health would remain pervasive in international mental health policy over the next three decades.

In the Diaspora

After 1973, Uganda ceased to be a major voice in international mental health. Most of the expatriate and many Ugandan psychiatrists left the country in the wake of Amin's expulsion of the Asian population in 1972. Those who remained did so in increasingly difficult circumstances, with little chance of being granted leave to attend international meetings or conferences. The loss of personnel, combined with political and economic insecurity, sent psychiatry into a long period of stagnation and decline, from which it would only start to recover in the 1990s. This drain on psychiatry in Uganda, however, coincided with the movement of psychiatrists into teaching, research and advisory positions elsewhere in Africa and beyond. Their movement highlights the increasing interconnectedness of international mental health, with practical experience—particularly 'on the ground' experience—being highly valued by universities and international organisations such as the WHO.

Those who sought an exit from the uncertainty and instability first of Amin's rule, and then the civil conflict that followed, found themselves in a privileged position compared to many others in Uganda. Following the leads of Uganda, Nigeria and Senegal, medical schools across Africa started investing in psychiatry, creating opportunities for psychiatrists to find work elsewhere. These psychiatrists took with them expertise in training as well as experience in research and public education. Joseph Muhangi, who had been promoted to Associate Professor and Head of the Department of Psychiatry after German's departure in 1972, was among those forced to look for opportunities elsewhere. Originating from Ankole and representing an educated elite, Muhangi was under threat of attack by Amin's forces, and when a new Senior Lectureship in Psychiatry was established at the University of Nairobi in 1975, he fled, taking what was most likely a significant cut in pay. In Nairobi, Muhangi introduced a new research programme in child psychiatry and helped to increase the allocation for psychiatry in the undergraduate medical curriculum from 200 to 300 hours. With his Kenyan colleague W. J. Muya, he drew up suggestions for the revision of the Mental Treatment Ordinance, last updated under colonial rule. With support from the University of Nairobi, Muhangi also continued to attend meetings of the Association of Psychiatrists in Africa, becoming Assistant-Editor-in-Chief of the newly established *African Journal of Psychiatry* in 1975.[52] In 1976, Muhangi was then joined by Wilson Acuda, a Ugandan psychiatrist who had been in London studying for the MrcPsych at the time of Amin's coup, and had been unable to return home. By the late 1970s, the increased number of staff at the Department of Psychiatry allowed the University of Nairobi to agree to postgraduate training, with a new MMed in Psychiatry, modelled on the Uganda syllabus.[53] In 1980, shortly after Amin's overthrow, Muhangi returned to Makerere, restarting the MMed programme and keen to rebuild psychiatry. Yet, like many others, Muhangi lived with 'enormous anger over what Amin had done'.[54] He turned to politics, running for and being elected an MP under Milton Obote's new government. A few months later, while travelling with his sons to visit family in Ankole, he was stopped and shot dead in front of his sons by anti-Obote guerrillas and left by the side of the road.[55] Acuda, meanwhile, stayed in Nairobi, becoming Professor and Head of the Department of Psychiatry in 1983. He then moved to Zimbabwe to head up the Department of Psychiatry, and in 1998 returned to the UK to work in the National Health Service (NHS), where he remained until retirement in 2012.[56]

The expatriate psychiatrists who left Uganda were even more mobile. John Cox returned to the UK, where he remained active within the fields of transcultural psychiatry and perinatal psychiatry, becoming Secretary General of the World Psychiatric Association (WPA), 2002–2008. He helped drive the agenda of British transcultural psychiatry on institutional racism, arguing for the dangers of making essentialist assumptions about race, culture and ethnicity in psychiatric training and practice.[57] Orley returned to the University of Oxford in 1973, before moving to the WHO's Division of Mental Health, Geneva, where he worked between 1983 and 1998, rising to become Programme Manager. In addition to work on all area's of the WHO's mental health programme, Orley was directly involved in formulating policy and guidelines on mental health in primary care, including *The Introduction of a Mental Health Component into Primary Health Care* (1990), which set out the 'practical steps' by which national governments might reorganise mental health services. He could easily have been speaking of his experience in Uganda when he noted in 1998 that the concept of primary health care arose 'in part as a reaction to the horrific inequalities that exist in medical care, in which a large proportion of the health budget goes towards a few specialist hospitals, usually teaching hospitals'.[58] Wood and German, meanwhile, both moved to Australia to take up positions there. German, from a new position at the University of Western Australia, continued to advise on mental health policy for the WHO Africa Regional Office and Western Pacific Region.[59] He returned to East Africa on multiple occasions in subsequent decades as a WHO consultant and, like Orley, he contributed to the further formulation of WHO policy on mental health in primary care. His contribution was given special mention in the preface to *The Introduction of a Mental Health Component into Primary Health Care* (1990).[60]

The global mobility afforded to psychiatry was not limited to psychiatrists, however. Vincent B. Wankiiri, one of the first psychiatric nurses, had observed the changes instituted by psychiatrists at Butabika Hospital, if he was critical of their refusal to embrace cultural ideas

and practices in treatment. He remained at Butabika through the
1970s but was offered an opportunity to travel by the WHO in the
early 1980s as a Psychiatric Nurse Tutor with postings in Lesotho,
Botswana and Swaziland as well as short-term training consultancies
elsewhere.[61] Like Uganda's psychiatrists, Wankiiri benefitted from the
value placed on practical experience, particularly in guiding national
governments towards community and primary health care approaches.
In Zimbabwe, he advised on the post-basic Psychiatric Nurse Training
Programme, aiming to bring it 'in line with current psychiatric nursing
approaches, including promotional, preventive and therapeutic mental
health care within the framework of primary health care'.[62] He contributed to the WHO Collaborative Study on Strategies for Extending
Mental Health Care being carried out in Brazil, Colombia, Egypt,
India, the Philippines, Senegal and Sudan and was a participating
investigator for the WHO's *Diagnostic and Management Guidelines for
Mental Disorders in Primary Care* (ICD-10 Chapter V, Primary Care
Version) (1996).[63]

Despite having complained about the lack of priority accorded to
psychiatry in Uganda, Wankiiri recalled how it was completely different in these countries: 'they didn't have anything, they didn't have any
psychiatrists', and where they did, they were of the 'old custodial care'
kind, 'and that's what I tried to break down by training nurses'.[64] His
were community mental health nurses, what he described as 'the modern care of psychiatric patients', and for whom Wankiiri helped develop
flow-charts for the identification and management of different mental
health problems.[65] He believed there could, and should, be an 'African'
model for mental health training, in which ideas of 'community' were
key, and where the only way to secure 'Health for All' was through collaboration between 'modern mental health care workers' and 'traditional
practitioners'.[66] Yet he encountered 'widespread negative attitudes' to
the use of community mental health nurses among key people, including, in Lesotho, 'some influential doctors at district hospitals' who were
themselves in charge of mental health units.[67] Those providing care to
the mentally ill were still regarded 'as custodians of "mad people"' and
some nurse managers preferred their nurses to spend time providing general nursing care in hospitals, 'rather than pay consultative visits to rural
health centres or visit patients' families'.[68] Wankiiri would spend the rest
of his career attempting to advocate for what he deemed to be a more
African-centric approach to mental health care.

CONCLUSION

From the early 1980s, mental health in primary care became a major plank of WHO policy on mental health. It remained in the shadow of the WHO's broader policy on primary health care, however. Despite the determination of WHO staff to raise of the profile of mental health during the early 1970s, it did not feature significantly in the WHO's 'Health for All by the Year 2000' resolution of 1977 or at the Alma-Ata International Conference on Primary Health Care in 1978. Hailed as 'a victory for international health at the community level',[69] the Declaration of Alma-Ata, which was signed by 175 countries, defined primary health care as 'essential health care based on practical, scientifically sound and socially acceptable methods and technology made universally accessible to individuals and families in the community through their full participation and at a cost that the community and country can afford to maintain at every stage of their development in the spirit of self-reliance and self-determination'.[70] It was to be an integral part of the national health system, aiming to bring 'health care as close as possible to where people live and work'.[71] Mental health was discussed at Alma-Ata but, significantly, was not included in the final declaration. This oversight had serious implications for those seeking funding for mental health programmes, and meant that not all countries included mental health within their definitions of primary health care in the years following the conference—Uganda included.[72] Only since the late 1990s, when the Uganda Government recognised an increase in mental health problems, has the Ministry of Health looked at ways to integrate mental health into primary health care through its National Mental Health Care Package. It remains a central irony within psychiatry in Uganda that it has needed to seek WHO advice on an approach that Uganda helped pioneer.[73]

The role of psychiatrists working in Africa during the late 1960s and early 1970s in shaping international mental health policy highlights the power of collective experience and shared knowledge during this moment of increased mobility and attention on the health problems of developing countries. While psychiatrists recognised variations in political, social, economic and cultural conditions, both within and between countries, they also saw common challenges and problems that required experimentation with such approaches as the use of psychiatric auxiliaries, group therapy, village settlements and rural psychiatric outpatient clinics. This was a period of innovation in mental health care across many developing countries, in which the WHO then sought out their guiding role. Following initial discussions on the organisation of mental health care, many of the psychiatrists who participated in regional and international conferences continued to seek out advocacy roles. In 1975, a more politically inclined Association of Psychiatrists in Africa changed its name to the Association of African Psychiatrists, reflecting both the increased number of indigenous-born psychiatrists on the continent as well as a desire for Observer status in the Organisation of African Unity (OAU). The notion of African psychiatrists having a unique perspective on the problems of mental illness in Africa was also reflected in the title of the Association's new *African Journal of Psychiatry*, of which Muhangi was Assistant Editor-in-Chief.[74]

In the longer term, however, African psychiatrists have contributed disproportionately little to research and policy within the field of international mental health. The Association of African Psychiatrists, along with its journal, collapsed in 1981 just as structural adjustment policies were starting to cripple health systems and universities, resulting in little time, funding and training for experiments or research. Reductions in travel allowances, combined with ongoing difficulties of staffing, have made it more difficult for psychiatrists to participate in conferences beyond national borders, and barriers to research and publication have resulted in relatively little research being published in international journals. While some psychiatrists continued to consult for the WHO, most did not, focusing on keeping psychiatry going within their own countries, often in difficult economic and political circumstances. Since the mid-1990s, most professional activity among psychiatrists has been limited to a regional sphere of influence. The Uganda Psychiatric Association has met for regular conferences since its formation in 1996. Psychiatrists in East Africa have met at annual scientific conferences since 1999, and a new and expanded African Association of Psychiatrists and Allied Professionals was formed in the early 2000s, starting with a meeting in Nairobi. Such activity, particularly since the early 2000s, suggests an important body of knowledge and experience that should play a central role in determining international, now global mental health policy, but which has nevertheless seen relatively little circulation outside of the continent.[75]

NOTES

1. N. Chorev, *The World Health Organization Between North and South* (Ithaca, 2012), p. 3
2. World Health Organization Archives (WHOA) M4/86/12(B) Jkt 1 (International Congresses of the World Federation of Mental Health), M. Pfister, 'Features and Trends in the Mental Health Work of the World Health Organization', 5 September 1961, p. 2.
3. Ibid.
4. World Health Organization, *The Role of Public Health Officers and General Practitioners in Mental Health Care: Eleventh Report of the Expert Committee on Mental Health* (Geneva, 1962).
5. World Health Organization, *Training of Psychiatrists: Twelfth Report of the Expert Committee on Mental Health* (Geneva, 1963).
6. Chorev, *The World Health Organization*, Ch. 3.
7. World Health Organization, *Organization of Mental Health Services in Developing Countries: Sixteenth Report of the WHO Expert Committee on Mental Health* (Geneva, 1975).
8. World Health Organization Library (WHOL) OMH/EC/74.11, N. Sartorius, 'Immediate Needs in Mental Health Services: A Note for Discussion', 22 October 1974, p. 1.
9. World Health Organization, *Organization of Mental Health Services in Developing Countries*.
10. *Mental Disorders and Mental Health in Africa South of the Sahara: CCTA/CSA-WFMH-WHO Meeting of Specialists on Mental Health* (Bukavu, 1958), p. 109.
11. M. M. Heaton, *Black Skin, White Coats: Nigerian Psychiatrists, Decolonization, and the Globalization of Psychiatry* (Ohio, 2013), p. 70.
12. G. I. Tewfik, 'Problems of Mental Illness in Uganda', in *Mental Disorders and Mental Health in Africa South of the Sahara: CCTA/CSA-WFMH-WHO Meeting of Specialists on Mental Health* (Bukavu, 1958), p. 62.
13. T. A. Lambo, ed., *First Pan-African Psychiatric Conference Report* (Ibadan, 1961).
14. G. A. German and A. C. Raman, 'From Birth to Maturity—Historical Aspects of the Association of Psychiatrists in Africa', *African Journal of Psychiatry* 2(2) (1976), p. 258.
15. Lambo, *First Pan-African Psychiatric Conference*, p. 264.
16. German and Raman, 'From Birth to Maturity', pp. 255–265.
17. Personal communication with G. A. German, 29 January 2012.
18. *Mental Health Services in the Developing World: Reports on Workshops on Mental Health, Edinburgh (1968) and Kampala (1969)*, Commonwealth Foundation Occasional Paper, IV (Hove, 1969).

19. German and Raman, 'From Birth to Maturity', p. 258.
20. *Mental Health Services in the Developing World*, p. 39.
21. Ibid., p. 35.
22. Ibid., pp. 35–36.
23. Ibid., p. 38.
24. Ibid., p. 36.
25. Ibid., p. 42.
26. Ibid.
27. Ibid.
28. G. M. Carstairs, 'Psychiatric Problems of Developing Countries', *The British Journal of Psychiatry* 123(574) (1973), p. 275.
29. *Mental Health Services in the Developing World*, p. 34.
30. WHOA NIE-HMD-002 Jkt 1 (Medical School, University of Ibadan), A. Boroffka, 'The Delivery of Mental Health Care', n.d., pp. 5–6.
31. *Mental Health Services in the Developing World*, p. 33.
32. Ibid., p. 34.
33. S. M. B. Diop, *The Place of Mental Health in the Development of Public Health Services*, Africa Regional Office (AFRO) Technical Papers no. 8 (Brazzaville, 1974), p. 32.
34. Diop, *The Place of Mental Health*, p. 7.
35. WHOL SEA/Ment./19 Annex 7, 'Recommendations of the International Workshop on Priorities in Mental Health Care (Held in Madurai, from 21 to 22 January 1971, under the Auspices of the World Federation for Mental Health)', p. 5.
36. WHOL OMH/EC/74.3, J. Moser, 'Approaches to the Development of Basic Mental Health Services', 1974, p. 1.
37. T. W. Harding, 'Introduction: Mental Health Services in the Developing Countries: The Issues Involved', in T. A. Baasher et al., eds., *Mental Health Services in Developing Countries: Papers Presented at a WHO Seminar on the Organization of Mental Health Services, Addis Ababa, 27 November–4 December 1973* (Geneva, 1975), p. 1.
38. WHOL OMH/74.3, J. Moser, 'Development of Mental Health Services in Africa', p. 7.
39. Harding, 'Introduction: Mental Health Services in the Developing Countries', p. 2.
40. WHOL OMH/74.3, Moser, 'Development of Mental Health Services in Africa'.
41. Harding, 'Introduction: Mental Health Services in the Developing Countries'.
42. Personal communication with German; *Proceedings of a Workshop on Alcohol and Drug Dependence of the Association of Psychiatrists in Africa* (Nairobi, 1974).

43. World Health Organization, *Organization of Mental Health Services in Developing Countries*.
44. Ibid., pp. 22–23.
45. Ibid., p. 32.
46. Ibid., p. 12.
47. R. Giel and T. W. Harding, 'Psychiatric Priorities in Developing Countries', *British Journal of Psychiatry* 128(6) (1976), pp. 513–522.
48. World Health Organization, *Mental Health Care in Developing Countries: A Critical Appraisal of Research Findings: Report of a WHO Study Group* (Geneva, 1984), p. 5.
49. World Health Organization, *Mental Health Care in Developing Countries*, p. 9.
50. N. Sartorius and T. W. Harding, 'The WHO Collaborative Study on Strategies for Extending Mental Health Care, I: The Genesis of the Study', *American Journal of Psychiatry* 140 (1984), pp. 1470–1473.
51. World Health Organization, *Mental Health Care in Developing Countries*, p. 54.
52. J. Muhangi, 'Psychiatry in Kenya: New Horizons in Medical Care', inaugural lecture delivered at the University of Nairobi, 31 January 1980.
53. Personal communication with W. Acuda, 21 October 2011.
54. Personal communication with German.
55. Personal communication with German.
56. Personal communication with Acuda.
57. D. Bhugra, 'Professor John Cox', *Psychiatric Bulletin* 27 (2003), p. 471; J. L. Cox, 'Cultural Psychiatry, Diversity and Political Correctness in a Shrinking World', *International Psychiatry* 5(2) (2008), pp. 27–28; Royal College of Psychiatrists, *Report of the Working Party to Review Psychiatric Practices and Training in a Multi-Ethnic Society*, Council Report CR48 (London, 1996).
58. J. Orley, 'Application of Promotion Principles', in *Preventing Mental Illness: Mental Health Promotion in Primary Care* (Chichester, 1998), p. 470.
59. Personal communication with German.
60. World Health Organization, *The Introduction of a Mental Health Component into Primary Health Care* (Geneva, 1990), p. 5.
61. Interview with V. Wankiiri (WAN-01), Kampala, 29 August 2011; WHOL AFR/MH/12, 'Training in Mental Health for Primary Health Care Workers'.
62. World Health Organization, *African Mental Health Action Group, Ninth Meeting, Geneva, 9 May 1986* (Geneva, 1986), p. 18.
63. T. Baasher et al., 'On Vagrancy and Psychosis', *Community Mental Health Journal* 19(1) (1983), pp. 27–41; World Health Organization, *Diagnostic and Management Guidelines for Mental Disorders in Primary Care: ICD-10 Chapter V Primary Care Version* (Göttingen, 1996).

64. Interview WAN-01.
65. WHOL AFR/MH/12, 'Training in Mental Health for Primary Health Care Workers', 1982.
66. [V.] B. Wankiiri, 'Problems in Achieving Mental Health for All in Southern Africa [Letter]', *World Health Forum* 12(2) (1991), p. 211.
67. V. B. Wankiiri, 'Delivering Mental Health Through Primary Health Care: The Lesotho Experience', *Epidemiology and Community Psychiatry* (Boston, 1985).
68. Wankiiri, 'Delivering Mental Health Through Primary Health Care'.
69. A.-E. Birn, 'The Stages of International (Global) Health: Histories of Success or Successes of History?' *Global Public Health: An International Journal for Research, Policy and Practice* 4(1) (2009), p. 58.
70. 'Declaration of Alma-Ata International Conference on Primary Health Care, Alma-Ata, USSR, 6–12 September 1978', http://www.who.int/publications/almaata_declaration_en.pdf, last accessed 23 February 2015.
71. M. Cueto, 'The Origins of Primary Health Care and Selective Primary Health Care', *American Journal of Public Health* 94(11) (2004), pp. 1864–1874; O. Gish, 'Selective Primary Care: Old Wine in New Bottles', *Social Science and Medicine* 16(10) (1982), pp. 1049–1054; J. E. Lawn et al., 'Alma-Ata 30 Years On: Revolutionary, Relevant, and Time to Revitalise', *Lancet* 372(9642) (September 2008), pp. 917–927; S. Litsios, 'The Long and Difficult Road to Alma-Ata: A Personal Reflection', *International Journal of Health Services* 32(4) (2002), pp. 709–732.
72. N. Sartorius, 'Mental Health and Primary Health Care', *Mental Health in Family Medicine* 5 (2008), p. 75.
73. Interview with S. Ndyanabangi (NDY-01), Ministry of Health, Kampala, 3 May 2011.
74. WHOA M4/86/25(4) (Fourth Pan African Psychiatric Congress, Abidjan, Ivory Coast, 30 June–5 July 1975), N. Sartorius, T. Harding, and J. Moser, 'Report on Attendance', n.d., p. 3.
75. O. Gureje and A. Alem, 'Hidden Science? A Glimpse at Some Work in Africa', *World Psychiatry* 3(3) (2004), pp. 178–181.

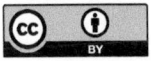

CHAPTER 7

The 'Trauma' of War and Violence

On 25 January 1971, Idi Amin and his army seized power in an apparently bloodless coup. Within a few minutes of the announcement on the radio, Kampala's streets were filled with crowds rejoicing the overthrow of President Milton Obote.[1] A large number of Makerere University students, too, joined in with celebrations in Buganda, having come to resent the violent and increasingly authoritarian nature of Obote's regime.[2] The initial optimism of Amin's coup, however, quickly faded as the realities of his rule became clear.[3] In the first year of the new regime, Amin's forces murdered several thousand Acholi and Langi soldiers suspected of disloyalty.[4] Soon after, Amin launched his 'economic war' against the 50,000 Ugandan Asians in the country, announcing the expulsion of these 'parasites' in August 1972.[5] The following months were characterised by a deteriorating security situation in which Amin's army and security services were allowed to kill with impunity, filling Uganda's prisons and torture centres—including the euphemistically named Public Safety Unit (PSU) and State Research Bureau (SRB)—with little or no regard for the law.[6]

Amin was ousted in April 1979 following the invasion from Tanzania of the Uganda National Liberation Front (UNLF) and the Tanzania Peoples' Defence Force (TPDF).[7] A series of short regimes followed—Yusuf Lule, Godfrey Binaisa and Paulo Muwanga—each attempting unity, but ultimately flawed in their attempts at reconciliation.[8] In elections in 1980 that were widely believed to have been rigged, Milton Obote and his Uganda

© The Author(s) 2019
Y. Pringle, *Psychiatry and Decolonisation in Uganda*,
Mental Health in Historical Perspective,
https://doi.org/10.1057/978-1-137-60095-0_7

People's Congress (UPC) returned to power in a regime popularly known as Obote II, pushing Uganda into a civil war that was likely more brutal and entailed more loss of life than had been the case under Amin. In the Luwero Triangle, an area to the north of Kampala, comprising Luwero, Mubende and Mpigi Districts, the government's counter-insurgency operations against Yoweri Museveni's National Resistance Army (NRA) involved massacres, torture, rape and famine.[9] It has been estimated that over 60% of civilians in the Luwero Triangle lost at least one first-degree relative.[10] As Leopold Tamale, a farmer from Mpigi District, explained to the Commission of Inquiry into Violations of Human Rights in 1989, 'there was no war', only a wanton killing of people.[11]

Obote was overthrown by Tito Okello and his army in July 1985. Refusing to negotiate with Okello, the NRA continued to fight, capturing Kampala in January 1986. By the time Museveni was sworn in as President on 29 January, Uganda had experienced fifteen years of violence and conflict. It has been estimated that over 600,000 people had been killed or 'disappeared', with a further 1.2 million refugees in neighbouring countries, including over 200,000 in southern Sudan (now South Sudan).[12] The installation of Museveni and his National Resistance Movement (NRM) government was not the end of internal conflict, however. Between 1986 and the early 2000s, violence continued in northern Uganda as the NRA attempted to pacify the remains of Okello's forces and numerous other guerrilla groups formed in response to NRA counter-insurgency operations. In the context of ongoing instability, a number of spirit mediums emerged, including Alice Auma (known also as Alice Lakwena), who with her Holy Spirit Battalion promised to cleanse Uganda, and Joseph Kony and his Lord's Resistance Army (LRA). Kony sought the moral rejuvenation of the Acholi people, becoming increasingly violent after the failure of peace talks with the government and Acholi elders in 1994, attacking many of the civilians he claimed to represent.[13] Over a million people were displaced either in an attempt to escape the LRA or as a result of counter-insurgency operations in the following years, prompting a major international humanitarian response. This has included emergency relief to internally displaced populations, peacebuilding programmes and, since the late 1990s, an upsurge in psychosocial programmes targeting both civilians and soldiers (particularly child soldiers). Since the early 2000s, humanitarian relief efforts in northern Uganda have come under fierce criticism for both exacerbating violence and undermining democratic processes.[14]

Psychiatry has provided a useful language for observers attempting to make sense of this period of Uganda's history, and the at times incomprehensible levels of violence. One of Amin's leading henchmen was Lieutenant Colonel Juma Ali, popularly known by civilians and military personnel as 'General Butabika'. In 1977, John Kibukamusoke, former Professor of Medicine at Mulago Hospital, a founder member of the National Association for Mental Health (NAMH) and one of Amin's personal physicians between 1971 and 1973, described to *The Observer* how Amin was almost certainly suffering from general paralysis of the insane (GPI), something that would explain his 'syndrome of grandiose paranoia', as well as 'hypomania', 'a state of mind in which a rapid succession of widely varying ideas hit the mind and receive oral expression'.[15] Caroline Lamwaka, a journalist who covered the war in northern Uganda, called Alice 'a lunatic prostitute turned witch'.[16] While Kony, lacking a clear political motive and using brutal tactics, has been variously declared 'mad', 'clinically insane', 'psychotic', 'delusional' and 'paranoid schizophrenic'.[17] Indeed, what else but madness to explain yet another case of apparently irrational African violence? What these explanations have lacked, however, is any attention to the ways in which these movements resonated with long-term upheavals and processes, or how brutality and fear could be seen as a rational means of exploiting a key resource—people.[18] A longer-term perspective, moreover, also raises questions about the legacies of a colonial state that legitimised the use of violence and which, in preparing for decolonisation, rapidly promoted soldiers and police officers through the policy of Africanisation.[19]

More pervasive than labels given to leaders, however, has been the use of psychiatric and psychologised language to define and describe populations 'traumatised' by violence. The civil war of the early 1980s, and the violence that continued in the north into the 1990s, coincided with a resurgence of interest in 'trauma' in Europe and the USA. In the USA, where Post-Traumatic Stress Disorder (PTSD) entered the Diagnostic and Statistical Manual of Mental Disorders III (DSM-III) in 1980, it was closely linked to the context of the Vietnam War. In Europe, it was tied to the 'collective remembering' of the Second World War, and particularly the Holocaust, with notions of 'collective trauma' being reborn in subsequent generations.[20] At a time when research on trauma was still in its infancy internationally, Uganda and Ugandan refugees became the subject of some of the earliest research on the psychological effects of war and violence in Africa. This focused at first on refugees and children rather than the broader population—two groups who could be regarded unambiguously as 'victims' in a conflict in which there were no clear 'sides'. It also did not elicit much by way of an immediate response from psychiatrists or humanitarian relief organisations. Barbara Harrell-Bond recalled the 'stiff resistance' of non-governmental organisations (NGOs) in northern Uganda and southern Sudan in the 1980s towards 'basic socio-psychological research' among refugee populations and little interest in 'designing interventions to mitigate the stresses associated with their experiences—violence, death and bereavement, uprooting, flight of the challenges of survival and adaptation in exile'.[21] By the late 1990s, however, psychosocial programmes, notably peer counselling, were occupying an increasingly important space within NGO and humanitarian activities, boosted by an upsurge of humanitarian activity following the Rwandan genocide in 1994, and the declaration of violence as a global public health issue by the World Health Organization (WHO) in 1996.[22] In 1998, the Uganda Government and UNICEF conducted a Northern Uganda Psycho-Social Needs Assessment, explaining that the population of Acholi, especially children, had witnessed 'psychologically wounding events'. An analysis of the psychological effects of war was deemed pertinent because the war had 'broken down the very fabric of civil society', and 'traditional customs which brought community people together to discuss problems and implement solutions jointly are no longer followed'.[23] In line with seeing violence as a public health issue, many of the subsequent programmes have been based on an underlying assumption that without help, traumatic experiences will lead to cycles of further violence.

This chapter, which explores the 'trauma' of war and violence in the 1980s and early 1990s, is included in this book because it highlights ways in which the decolonisation of psychiatry remained incomplete. While psychiatric services continued to be underfunded and of little relevance to most in the face of war and violence, psychosocial activities, driven primarily by international agencies and specialists, attracted significant amounts of attention and money. And while many of these activities have increasingly been appropriated by the Ugandans who were trained to run them, the creation of knowledge about trauma was driven for a long time by expatriate psychiatrists, with their own interests in culture, suffering and victimhood. In assessments of the psychological effects of war and violence in the 1980s and early 1990s, Uganda's psychiatrists were largely absent. This is hardly surprising considering that psychiatric services were on the brink of almost complete collapse after well over a decade of political and economic insecurity. Continuing to offer even the most basic psychiatric services in these conditions took priority over concern about 'trauma'. But this was not without criticism, particularly from a new generation of psychiatrists. In 1992, trainee psychiatrist James Edward Walugembe challenged his colleagues at Mulago Hospital to think about why, despite over twenty-five years of civil war and violence, they were not even thinking about PTSD.[24] As Walugembe posited, there was a problem in research on trauma being directed by a range of international 'experts', rather than Ugandan psychiatrists, it being more humanitarian than psychiatric in nature.

DECLINE AND STAGNATION

In February 1971, James Namakajo, formerly a press officer with Obote's Ministry of Information, then a speech-writer to Amin, was arrested and confined in Makindye Military Barracks. Amin claimed, when asked by Ali Mazrui, then Professor of Political Science at Makerere University, that Namakajo had been found on the Fourth Floor of the President's Office with a pistol, intending to kill him. While he was not held in the 'Singapore' cell of Makindye, a place where 'you had no chance of return', Namakajo and his friends feared for his life. Shortly after his confinement, Namakajo recalled, a friend arranged for their father, a doctor, to visit him in Makindye and 'write a recommendation that I was mentally disturbed and take me to Butabika so that I could escape death'. Psychiatry, in this instance, provided a potential means of safety, regarded as superior to conditions within military barracks. The plan failed, but Namakajo was able to secure a transfer to a prison with better conditions shortly after, and was released within a month, his favour having been restored with a temperamental Amin.[25]

Even if there had been the will among psychiatrists and others to use psychiatry to subvert political action, psychiatry did not have the power to be effective. Between 1972 and 1982, the Ministry of Health's real expenditure per head of population was estimated by the World Bank to have fallen by eighty-five per cent.[26] Medical staff fled the country or sought alternative employment in private practice, as salaries eroded under inflation and working conditions deteriorated. By the mid-1980s, Butabika Hospital was operating at a third of capacity (approximately 300 patients), lacking transport, electricity, an adequate water supply or sewerage system, sufficient staff numbers, money for food or drugs, equipment for the Occupational Rehabilitation Unit, or funds to bury dead bodies outside of hospital grounds.[27] In 1987, the World Health Organization (WHO) country representative for Uganda sent a long list of 'urgent requirements' to the African Mental Health Action Group. This included emergency relief supplies of drugs, stationery and commodities for patients, rehabilitation of infrastructure, decentralisation and integration of mental health into primary care, recruitment and training of more personnel, provision of books, journals and transport, strategies for monitoring and evaluating mental health services, and 'a clearly defined mental health policy and programme for the country'.[28] As G. G. C. Rwegellera, Lecturer in Psychiatry, remarked in 1986, 'what is left now is nothing but a shadow of what was once a reasonably good and growing psychiatric care delivery system'.[29]

The Department of Psychiatry was almost immediately affected by the insecurity of Amin's regime following his coup in 1971. G. Allen German recalled being asked by the British High Commission to be their daily telephone contact at Makerere University, charged with providing security advice to British families working at the university. 'No doubt Amin's forces were monitoring my phone', German described: 'I don't know for sure—but I became aware that I was being followed...I was then detained and accused of being a British spy. Detention was unpleasant but mercifully brief'.[30] In the intervening period, all British clinical staff at Makerere Medical School were warned, via a television broadcast, that they 'had been acting against him [Amin]' and were advised to leave.[31] Many of those working in the Department of Psychiatry left in the following months, whether because of the decree expelling Ugandan Asians, or because they feared for their own safety. Lovette Coelho, the Departmental Secretary, was among those forced to leave. German's wife, moreover, as a Seychellois, was regarded by the Amin regime as Asian, and so, 'with some anxiety', German set about making their own preparations. On hearing this news, German recalled, Stephen Bosa attempted to intervene, putting 'his life and security at risk in so doing. His approaches were rebuffed'.[32] By the beginning of 1974, Klaus Minde, John Cox, F. J. Harris, John Orley and Harry Egdell had also left the country, the WHO-funded lectureship was vacant, and Wilson Acuda, who had been studying at the Institute of Psychiatry in London in April 1972, was unable to return due to the political situation.[33] Joseph Muhangi, fearing for his life, followed in 1975 by moving to the

University of Nairobi. Such was the shortage of psychiatrists that Bosa, who was due to retire from government service at the end of 1972, was re-engaged on local contract terms as a Senior Consultant (Psychiatrist) in March 1973 on the personal request of Amin and the Ministry of Health.[34]

With the exodus of psychiatrists, the National Association for Mental Health (NAMH) and the Mental Health Advisory Committee (MHAC) ceased to exist. At least one new group was formed in their absence, however, using Jinja Hospital as a base. In 1973, Peter Matovu, one of the first Psychiatric Social Workers (PSWs) trained under the scheme devised by Harris, and finally recognised by the Ministry of Health, organised a Busoga Psychiatric Advisory Committee. It included among its members a psychiatrist from Butabika Hospital, physicians and nurses from Jinja Hospital, and representatives from the police, prison, probation service and Church of Uganda. The small mental health clinic at Jinja, established by E. B. Ssekabembe in 1970, provided official justification for the group in a context where any meeting was looked upon with suspicion. Topics included problems of insufficient accommodation for mental patients at Jinja Hospital, severe staff shortages, language problems, as well as the lack of transport for follow-up visits.[35] In addition, it sought to continue the mental health promotion activities of the NAMH, publishing articles on mental illness in the *Voice of Uganda*. Ongoing problems caused by stereotypes of the mentally ill were at the fore, not least among members of the Committee itself, who had to be asked not to use outdated terms such as 'lunatic', assume that it was common for patients to pretend to be mentally ill, or that those trying to help might be 'hunted by patients...citing a well known example where this almost happened'.[36]

Where psychiatry continued at Butabika and Makerere it did so because of the determination of those involved. A. M. Kitumba, who had been in London completing the Diploma in Psychological Medicine (DPM), returned to Uganda after 1972 and replaced J. W. Kasirye as Medical Superintendent of Butabika Hospital. In increasingly trying circumstances, Kitumba and Bosa were left to steer psychiatric services almost single-handedly. Kitumba kept up a regular stream of requests to the Ministry of Health and other government departments for maintenance, repair and improvement works at Butabika, while Bosa, exhibiting his usual stubbornness in the face of difficult circumstances, continued to consult with patients.[37] When, due to the absence of transport and security, staff at Mulago Hospital Mental Health Clinic abandoned their positions, Bosa's response was to camp in the wards with several days' food for the inpatients and himself.[38] Such was his determination, according to his eldest son, that one day, 'medical students seeing him walk rather than drive into hospital (he had a house half a kilometer away) cheered him and said "Eh, Professor, you are walking on feet!" to which he replied, "Thank God I am not walking on my head."'[39] In 1975, Bosa returned to Makerere Medical School to take over teaching in psychiatry, and in 1979 convinced the Ministry of Health to set up a Psychiatric Clinical Officers (PCO) Training School at Butabika Hospital. Bosa returned to Butabika in 1987 to launch the new training programme but here, age and longer-term difficulties with hierarchy reappeared. By 1988, staff at Butabika Hospital complained that Bosa had lost interest in visiting patients and, in their opinion, 'stopped working for the Government years ago'.[40]

The training programmes initiated by Bosa were small in scale if not in ambition. The PCO Training School started with six students, trained in practical and theoretical psychiatry over two years, with the ultimate aim that each district might have at least two PCOs to serve them. By 1988, the school remained 'an improvised one', with no formal building,[41] but had trained a handful of new PCO officers, including Silver K. Kasoro, who was posted to Fort Portal, Kabarole District, in western Uganda.[42] At Makerere, moreover, Fred N. Kigozi was the first to complete the relaunched MMed in 1979, followed in 1980 by Grace Nakasi, Uganda's first female psychiatrist. In 1981, Emilio Ovuga, from a remote corner of north-western Uganda, completed the MMed but, due to the civil war, immediately left for positions in Kenya and South Africa, only returning to the Department of Psychiatry in 1989.[43] Florence Baingana, who submitted a dissertation on patient views of traditional healers in 1987, completed the MMed in 1990.[44] Having both worked at Butabika since the mid-1980s, Margaret Mungherera and David Basangwa similarly passed the MMed in Psychiatry in 1992 and 1994, respectively.[45] As a result of the new training schemes, there were five psychiatrists in either government or university service by 1987. With all based in Kampala, the number was inadequate, but was nevertheless essential in preventing the complete collapse of psychiatry in the subsequent decade.

By the late 1980s, the effects of insecurity and financial mismanagement on psychiatry were painfully clear. There had been no renovations to the buildings for over ten years, most of the wards had no mattresses and were 'in total darkness' at night, and a lack of food meant that Butabika Hospital staff who had not left for better working conditions elsewhere were struggling to feed patients more than once a day.[46] The hospital remained financially dependent on the Ministry of Health, receiving significantly less than other hospitals, relative to size.[47] More worrying for the reputation of psychiatry among the general public was the lack of security. Broken locks and windows in the wards, as well as a lack of fencing, meant that only a few hours after admission, relatives were finding their patients roaming the streets of Kampala. In one incident in 1987, a patient walked out of the male admission ward and caused 'grievous damage to a baby in the next village'.[48] Fears about safety, which had a long history in Uganda, also compounded the low status of psychiatry in relation to other medical disciplines, making it difficult to attract staff. On hearing that he had been asked to take up the position of Medical Superintendent at Butabika in 1987, relieving Kitumba of administrative responsibility, Ben Kawooya recalled how 'Learned friends of mine genuinely tried to persuade me not to move from Mulago to Butabika. One said it was a demotion....Another one burst out laughing and warned me to take care. It wasn't safe what with all those madmen'.[49]

Those in charge of Butabika in the late 1980s and early 1990s argued that 'bias ignorance' against psychiatry and chronic underfunding were preventing psychiatry from recovering.[50] Yet infighting between those in management roles was likely also exacerbating the situation. A Ministry of Health inspector to Butabika Hospital in 1991 issued a damning report highlighting problems relating to leadership, financial management, staffing, training, patient records and patient care. By this point, the hospital had only three active doctors and a payroll that was heavily bloated by 'ghost workers'—the dead, absentees and fictitious staff who all drew a regular salary. The remaining staff were 'poorly motivated', taking part in 'excessive pilfrage [sic.] of hospital property', and demoralised by meagre salaries and poor working conditions. As a result of vandalism during the civil war, there were still no beds for patients, no bedding, drugs, electricity or running water, locks or window panes, or suitable kitchen facilities. Patient services were 'at the brink of collapse', and those at Butabika were now almost completely isolated from Kampala, with the road network destroyed and the hospital transport system 'virtually grounded'. The records system was also non-existent, it not being unusual for patients to be admitted and discharged without any proper medical records being kept. Yet as the inspector made clear, the situation at Butabika Hospital was 'not Butabika's problem alone', but rather 'a prototype of what is happening elsewhere' in general hospitals and clinics.[51] Restructuring and new leadership needed to be at the heart of rehabilitation.

The stagnation and pessimism surrounding psychiatry during the 1980s and early 1990s was reflective of the wider irrelevance of psychiatry within Uganda. In contrast to psychiatry's involvement in discourses of national development during the 1960s, psychiatrists remained absent from national discussions about economic and social recovery until well into the 1990s. Psychiatry also had little to offer those affected by war and violence. Traditional healing flourished during the 1980s, with only the smallest minority of people exhibiting mental distress eventually reaching Butabika. Into the gap left by psychiatry, however, came a primarily externally driven, donor-funded concern for the psychological effects of war and violence, which has been more humanitarian than psychiatric in practice and delivery, and which privileged the pursuit of knowledge of collective populations.

In Search of 'War Trauma'

Refugees started crossing the border from Uganda into Sudan in mid-1979, fearing for their physical safety and livelihoods. Numbers were small at first, following the UNLF and the TPDF's invasion of Uganda. They then grew considerably after the fall of Amin's regime, particularly when the newly formed NLA prevented national elections in 1980 and launched a war of revenge on the ethnic groups most closely associated with Amin's government. In March 1982, the number of assisted refugees in settlements and transit camps in southern Sudan was approximately 9000. By September 1983, it had reached 95,000.[52] The emergency assistance programme launched in response included United Nations High Commissioner for Refugees (UNHCR), the Sudan Government's office of the Commission for Refugees (COMREF), and numerous NGOs and international voluntary agencies, including Norwegian Church Aid, the Africa Committee for Rehabilitation of Southern Sudan (ACROSS), the Southern Sudan Rehabilitation Assistance Project (SSRAP), OXFAM and Médecins Sans Frontières (MSF). These organisations were little interested in the mental health of African refugees, seeing even basic socio-psychological research as a neglect of humanitarian duties.[53] When a psychiatrist from Juba Hospital, Sudan, approached UNHCR in 1979, stating that those arriving might have special health needs and offering to survey the problem, his offer was declined.[54] 'Refugees', Harrell-Bond noted following field-work in Yei River District in 1982–1983, 'are expected to cope by being appropriately "social", but they are denied the resources to re-establish the real bases of social life', customs that required money, food and livestock to pay bridewealth, conduct burial rites and host funerals.[55] In the absence of psychological or psychiatric assistance for individual cases, responses to distress frequently involved either ignoring those who came to their offices, or handing out Valium indiscriminately.[56] Moses D., a 34-year-old former soldier and prisoner of war, had arrived in Sudan as a refugee in late 1982. He had been tortured and had spent a short period at Butabika Hospital for mental treatment as a result.[57] Soon after his arrival in Sudan, he sought medical assistance, first at Yei, then at Juba Hospital, where it was decided that he should go to Khartoum for more specialist treatment. The international humanitarian German Medical Team, however, disagreed with this decision and sent him back to his refugee camp. In an attempt to overturn the decision, Moses D. appealed to UNHCR and returned to Juba Hospital and the German Medical Team office. However, now labelled as a 'psychiatric case', he reported being treated as an extreme annoyance: 'I was surprised to see the doctor of GMT [German Medical Team] very angry...He tore the letter of the doctor of the regional hospital to pieces and asked me to leave immediately....When I went they promised to have no more dealings with me'.[58] Relief workers were poorly trained, and limited resources and time meant there was no incentive for dealing with refugees as individuals.[59]

Harrell-Bond had not set out to conduct research on the mental health problems of refugees. She stressed that she had 'actually resisted facing the possibility that African refugees might share such problems with other refugees about whom I had read', most likely referring to refugees on the Thai-Cambodian border. Yet she also pointed to her 'unrealistic and naive faith in the power of the family system to buffer individuals undergoing stress'—the assumption, reminiscent of colonial psychiatry, that Africans shared common ideas and practices that provided stabilising influences, something that Harrell-Bond called an 'over-socialised concept of man'.[60] While maintaining that 'economical explanations' were at the heart of much of the 'abnormal social behaviour' she observed in southern Sudan, 'serious attention' to psychosocial issues was 'long overdue'.[61] On her request, Alex de Waal and Alula Pankhurst, colleagues from the University of Oxford, travelled to southern Sudan in 1984. With three Ugandan colleagues they administered a Present State Examination (PSE), an interview technique that originated in the work of John K. Wing, of the Institute of Psychiatry, London, on how psychiatrists could describe, record and categorise the symptoms of schizophrenia. By the early 1980s, the PSE had been used in numerous cross-cultural studies of mental illness, based on, and also confirming, the dominant assumption in cross-cultural psychiatry that mental illness categories were universal. De Waal and Pankhurst justified their use of the PSE among refugees in southern Sudan by reference to this wider body of collective knowledge, using a modified version of an already 'cross-culturally validated' PSE administered by Orley in Uganda in a study published with Wing in 1979.[62]

The team conducted at least fifty-seven interviews, which were then analysed by clinical psychologists in Oxford. Of these, three-quarters showed an 'appreciable psychiatric disorder', notably anxiety and depression.[63] In contrast to cases of anxiety and depression in Europeans, their respondents presented primarily somatic symptoms, including headaches, aches, exhaustion, sleeplessness and loss of appetite.[64] The study had some major flaws, recognised by those involved, including a small sample size. More significant was the inexperience of the interview team, which might have meant they had difficulty differentiating between emotional states, or potentially have confused terms for 'depression' and 'annoyance', which in Luganda at least were to a certain extent interchangeable.[65] The researchers nevertheless concluded that the potential incidence of psychological distress and psychiatric illness was relatively high among refugees in southern Sudan. This did not necessarily mean that psychiatry or counselling was required, but rather represented a call for further research and for humanitarian aid programmes to consider mental health as a priority. The language of PTSD and 'war trauma' had been absent. Instead, they had been concerned more generally with anxiety, depression and stress arising from not only from conflict but from life as a refugee. Through this, Harrell-Bond was making a wider point about the failure of relief workers to consider refugees as individuals with their own social and political histories, or even to consult assisted refugees about the kinds of assistance that would be most beneficial to them. The irony of administering a PSE to gather 'indirect evidence' for psychological distress among refugees was perhaps lost here.

The use of research to advocate for the development of humanitarian interventions also lay behind the purpose of a series of investigations on war and 'child stress' in 1985–1986. Led by Cole P. Dodge, UNICEF representative in Uganda since 1981, and Magne Raundalen, a Norwegian psychologist, their collaborators included James Lwanga, Lecturer in Psychiatry at Makerere University, Charles Mugisha, a paediatrician at the Nutrition Centre, Makerere University, and Atle Dyregrove, a psychologist with expertise in disaster, grief and stress research. While not formally sponsored by UNICEF, the investigations nevertheless aimed to provide a basis for developing intervention strategies with parents, relief workers, teachers, health professionals and government—'to advocate the children's cause more strongly, especially with regard to their protection during times of war, violence and extreme stress'.[66] They represented the first investigations into children's reactions to war in Africa, providing opportunities to gain 'more valid knowledge transculturally' through comparisons with studies of children exposed to 'war stress' in Europe during the Second World War, the Yom Kippur war, Cambodia and Northern Ireland.[67]

Due to insecurity across most of the country, the research was limited to the relative safety of Kampala. It comprised four interrelated investigations: the researchers asked 450 13–15-year-olds to write essays on the topics of 'War and violence in my life', 'The story of my life' and 'Events that made me happy and events that made me sad', they conducted 297 interviews of children's experiences of war and collected 40 compositions from 13–18-year-olds during the first week after the coup of 27 July 1985.[68] A doctor and clinical psychologist also interviewed 79 displaced children from the Luwero Triangle, now living in a Red Cross shelter. The clinical psychologist declared that 80% of these children had signs of depression of which most, unsurprisingly, were 'probably due to the experienced loss of home and close relatives'. Using language that the children themselves may not have used, the researchers described how children spoke of 'running desperately and experiencing extreme anxiety', summarising their descriptions with the word 'horror'.[69] What was most concerning for the researchers was that most appeared to have 'dissociated themselves from strong emotional responses', describing 'the horrible events without accompanying feelings'.[70] Basing their conclusions on research on trauma in Europe, this 'growing a shell' was 'a sign of highly traumatized children who have had little or no opportunity of working through emotionally what they have experienced'.[71] Children, along with refugees and internally displaced populations, were not only relatively accessible populations for research into the psychological effects of war and violence, but represented groups whose suffering could be declared unambiguously. This was particularly the case with children living in the Red Cross shelter. The researchers not only presumed that the children had similar backgrounds which might allow for useful comparisons but, after expressing some concern that their experiences might make them 'students of war', stressed that they were, clearly, 'victims of war'.[72]

In the years following the civil war of the early 1980s, another group which was able to mobilise international support was that of 'victims of torture'. The call for assistance had originated with the Nairobi branch of Amnesty International, which had asked two British doctors in 1985 to examine sixteen Ugandans who reported sexual violence, beatings, being burnt, and starvation. One of these, Elizabeth Gordon, a consultant surgeon with ten years experience examining torture victims, stated publicly that 'I have never seen such gross mutilations as I saw on these Ugandans'.[73] In response, the London-based Medical Foundation for the Care of Victims of Torture (now Freedom from Torture) contacted Patrick Bracken, a psychiatrist, and Joan E. Giller, a gynaecologist then working with Karen refugees on the Thai-Burmese border, proposing that they set up a centre offering physical and psychological support for victims of torture in Uganda. The centre was to be based on the model provided by existing centres in London, Canada, Norway, and Denmark, where victims of torture had been subject to medical and psychological investigation and rehabilitation programmes since the early 1980s.[74] Recalling the request, Giller stressed that she had felt uncomfortable with the 'assumptions and expectations of being the expert' in Thailand, knowing little about tropical medicine or work in resource-poor contexts, her very presence having a silencing effect on local knowledge. Uganda, by contrast, seemingly represented something different, 'a project which seemed, on the face of it, so clear-cut and unambiguous'.[75] In practice, this was far from the case. First was their location in Kampala, where the team arrived to set up the Medical Foundation (Uganda) in 1987. Like other Kampala-based institutions, this was largely inaccessible to most of the population, and far remote from those areas still affected by conflict. Resentment was already forming against international NGOs who were '"parachuting in" large numbers of expatriate staff living in relative comfort in Kampala dispensing largess', with only three of over sixty NGOs in the country working in northern Uganda.[76] Second, the category of 'victims of torture' was highly problematic in a context in which most people had witnessed atrocities and were now living in poverty or 'extreme physical hardship'.[77] To focus on those who had been tortured during periods of detention was to elevate their needs over others, based solely on the agenda of the international organisation providing the funding. The differing expectations of those who did visit the centre quickly made this clear. As Bracken and Giller reflected: people asked for material assistance, basic medication such as drugs for malaria, or work; the only thing 'that no one asked for was any form of psychological assistance'.[78] To continue to focus their efforts on the centre 'would have been to commit one of the worst crimes of which colonialism, and now neo-colonialism, has been guilty: to undermine local knowledge and local ways of doing things in favour of interventions of often dubious efficacy'.[79]

Abandoning the category of 'torture-victim', Bracken and Giller broadened their work to include psychological and physical support for those affected by violence in the Luwero Triangle but which, in practice, was still shaped by their own interests and expertise. Giller operated a travelling clinic for women who had been raped, offering physical examinations, including an HIV test for those who wanted it, as well as support groups facilitated by a social worker, Stella Kabaganda. In one meeting, a woman exclaimed 'with her arm in the air': 'Who amongst us has not been raped?', and received 'cries of approval' for her call. 'It felt as though a floodgate of emotion had been opened', Giller noted, 'and we were warmly welcomed and encouraged in what we proposed to do'. Yet, as in Kampala, when they brought up the idea of counselling, no one requested it. Instead, 'They wanted advice, medication, practical and financial assistance and reassurance'.[80] Bracken, meanwhile, turned towards research, undertaking a survey of the psychological effects of violence in the Luwero Triangle. In doing so, Bracken hoped to produce knowledge that would not only shape humanitarian and health worker priorities in Uganda, but would have relevance for humanitarian assistance in conflict and post-conflict settings elsewhere. This included questioning the cross-cultural validity of psychological instruments related to PTSD (which he nevertheless used during his own survey), as well as the assumption that psychotherapy was the most appropriate means of dealing with psychological disturbance relating to war. Not only did Bracken find that 'there was no great increase in severe psychiatric breakdown' and less psychological disturbance than expected, but 'The distress associated with trauma...[was]...often not conceptualised as a medical problem, and local family networks and traditional healers...[were]...felt to be the appropriate agents to deal with it'.[81]

By the time Bracken, Giller and Kabaganda published their first publicly accessible report on their work in 1992, they held up their work with victims of violence in Uganda as a mistake overcome, with lessons to be learned from the original highly centralised approach and the privileging of Western concepts and knowledge about trauma and PTSD.[82] With Derek Summerfield, Bracken and Giller would go on to present radical critiques of the assumptions underlying the proliferation of programmes providing mental health care for refugees and victims of violence, particularly in developing countries. They criticised the modernist agenda of reducing suffering to standardised measurements, the ethical issues of authenticating a particular type of victimhood and the treatment of 'trauma' as something to be discovered and managed by Western professionals.[83] In spite of this, as the number of NGOs and humanitarian agencies grew significantly in Uganda during the 1990s, both in response to the intensification of violence in northern Uganda after 1994, and in the use of Uganda as a base from which to address other conflicts in the Great Lakes region, these criticisms would pass many by.[84]

Research on the psychological effects of war and violence continued into the 1990s, spurred by high-level interest in violence by the UN and the provision of the first significant amounts of funding for research on violence by international organisations. Research in Uganda focused, again, on well-defined and accessible populations, aiming to produce methodologically rigorous data that could be compared with other conflict and post-conflict settings. Refugee camps in northern Uganda and southern Sudan in particular offered a unique opportunity to embark on a long-term research project on psychosocial programmes in post-conflict contexts, with approximately 250,000 Sudanese refugees accessible to the researchers in Moro and Arua Districts.[85] The camps housing these refugees represented what many assumed (wrongly) to be depoliticised spaces, with no serious attention paid to the ongoing violence of the refugee camps themselves.[86] From 1991, Uganda was part of a cross-cultural study on the psychosocial and mental health problems of refugees and victims of organised violence, a collaboration between the Netherlands government-funded International Institute for Psychosocial and Socio-Ecological Research (IPSER), the WHO and the World Federation for Mental Health (WFMH). The aim of the study, which also included Mozambique, Ethiopia, Cambodia and Tibetans in exile in India, was to use simple screening procedures to determine psychological morbidity, investigate the psychological problems encountered by refugees, develop and test training modules and materials for counsellors, to train trainers, and to evaluate all aspects of the project.[87] In Uganda, not only was psychosocial support required 'from a human point of view', but it was hoped that it would 'stimulate economic reconstruction'.[88] The activities involved training trainers who had histories as refugees, as well as providing training for twenty counsellors, psychiatric nurses, pastoral workers, medical assistants, female community leaders, primary school teachers and at least seventeen traditional healers.[89] It was hoped that this would enable those trained 'to recognize children and adults suffering from the consequences of trauma', to provide psychosocial support by setting up self-help groups, and by referring individuals to mental health professionals, where necessary.[90] According to the project lead, J. T. V. M. de Jong, the psychosocial approach was necessary not because of any conclusions drawn from existing research, but because the scale of suffering meant that it was impossible to address trauma through crisis intervention by psychiatrists and psychologists. Instead, a public mental health approach based on community action was necessary.[91]

While Ugandans were trained to conduct research and lead psychosocial support programmes, programmes which they undoubtedly adapted and shaped, research on the psychological effects of war and violence remained in the hands of international organisations and researchers. It was in direct response to this ongoing dominance of international 'expertise' that in 1992, Walugembe, then enrolled on the MMed in Psychiatry, screened new admissions at Mulago Mental Health Clinic for PTSD. While Walugembe argued that more attention needed to be paid to the cultural manifestations of PTSD in Africa, he stressed that the diagnosis was universal. If international researchers were looking for trauma, then it was the duty of Ugandan psychiatrists to at least screen for PTSD, and to conduct their own research into the cross-cultural applicability of the diagnosis. Acknowledging the limitations of his small sample size (100 patients), Walugembe argued that 24% of patients met the DSM-III-R criteria for a diagnosis of PTSD, with a further 11%, who did not meet the criteria, also reporting experiencing a serious traumatic event associated with war. He challenged his colleagues at Mulago to ask why, after over twenty-five years of war and violence, which included 'panda gari' ('pick me up' detainee screening) operations, psychiatrists at Mulago Mental Health Clinic were not diagnosing cases of PTSD. Yet, he acknowledged, people remained reluctant to visit psychiatrists. For Walugembe, this was not due to the ongoing irrelevance of psychiatry (though that was part of it), but because coping with trauma was something that people turned to traditional healers and their communities for support.[92]

COPING WITH WAR

Many international visitors to Uganda in the late 1980s and early 1990s arrived with assumptions that they would find whole populations 'traumatised' by war and violence. Amelia Brett, a social worker who visited in March 1991 following a gap of sixteen years, reflected that she had 'expected to find evidence of psychological damage'. What she found, however, 'was the energy, positiveness and will to rebuild shattered lives'.[93] Giller, moreover, noted that despite reading widely about Uganda, 'we knew so little about Ugandan people and how they appeared to be coping in the aftermath of tragedy without the aid of therapist or counsellor'.[94] What emerged from these observations was an intense interest in culturally and socially sanctioned modes of healing which, it was assumed, were playing a vital psychological role. According to Giller, this interest came as a surprise to many Ugandan health and medical practitioners, something she put down to Western medicine having 'instilled a sense of shame with respect to traditional healing', and a legacy of colonialism which had 'undermined any sense of worth in traditional ways of doing things',[95] but which perhaps also needs to be seen in the context of longer professional struggles for authority in the management of illness and health. Health and medical syllabi were still dominated by Western medical concepts, particularly with regard to psychiatry and psychology, and there was little place for traditional medicine in 'modern' practice.

Accounts of a resurgence of traditional medicine can be found across Uganda and southern Sudan, particularly in light of the decline of health, medical and social welfare systems. Herbalists were active in assisted refugee camps in southern Sudan in the early 1980s, providing, beyond the Valium offered by UNHCR, the only therapeutic option for those with mental illness.[96] Visitors to the Luwero Triangle in the years after the end of the civil war reported a 'flourishing' of traditional healing, including well-attended and regular healing ceremonies. Traditional healers, according to Bracken, were 'playing a double role'. Not only were they providing therapy to individuals in a context where the health and medical infrastructure had been destroyed, but they 'functioned as an important link with the past and thus contributed to a sense of continuity in a community which had just endured a very violent onslaught on its way of life'.[97] Traditional healers reported seeing more cases of *eddalu* (madness), *obusiru* (foolishness) and *akalogojjo* (a mild form of mental illness, characterised by confusion) since the war, but they had also seen increases in a wide range of physical illnesses, something they attributed to poor living conditions and dirty water causing an imbalance in the body. Significantly, in the context of international interest in the topic, they did not recognise a specific category of those suffering from 'war trauma'.[98]

More informal community and church-based networks, where they remained intact, may have provided an alternative form of support. At the opening of a new handpump in Luwero three months after the end of the civil war, teachers and clergy organised several hundred children into an hour-long dance portraying the history of the war, including well-known local incidents and solo performances from children who recounted their own experiences.[99] In another case, a 45-year-old man, who had had both his hands cut off by soldiers in the Luwero Triangle, was now almost entirely reliant on neighbours for assistance. While he continued to face practical difficulties, he reported that 'the support and solidarity shown...by his neighbours had allowed him to return to a fairly normal life'.[100] In March 1986, a fifteen-year-old girl who had until that point not been able to talk with her parents about being abducted and raped by UNLA soldiers, recounted her experiences in front of a small congregation in a Catholic Church in Nakaseki, Kampala. Regarded as a form of therapeutic cleansing, the girl was committing herself to God, and preparing to become a nun.[101] In a transit camp in northern Uganda, moreover, counsellors reported that there were 'almost weekly dancing sessions during which people sing traditional songs, including ones in which they introduce their miserable experiences'. The call of the drums would, according to the counsellors, bring people from all over the camp, with people 'recognizing their clan by the sound of the drums'.[102] As a result of such reports, the organisers of the IPSER-WHO-WFMH collaborative study noted their desire to do more to draw on 'indigenous coping strategies and culturally mediated protective factors'.[103] Counsellors were already using prayer to conclude group sessions, but more needed to be done to take 'a community-based mental health care approach and adapt the methods of counselling taking the context of the local culture into account'.[104]

Such accounts of culturally and socially mediated forms of healing and support only reinforce the marginality of the existing psychiatric system. One patient attending Mulago Mental Health Clinic in 1993 was a male soldier from Luwero District, who refused to discuss his combat experience, but described being ambushed by guerrillas, seeing friends killed, and feeling obliged to fight for the rebel side. Having lost all his relatives by the end of the war, he decided to join the regular army, where he subsequently lost his leg. He reported having 'frequent nightmares related to combat' and, according to Walugembe, met the clinical definition for PTSD. But the patient did not believe that psychiatry could help him. Instead, he wanted 'at least a 6 months leave to go and perform the cleansing ritual to get rid of the spirits of the people he had killed, whom he believed were haunting him and keeping him tense and awake all the time'.[105] In a similar case, a sixteen-year-old boy had joined the army after his father was killed by a rebel group and, after months of 'active combat', had been injured during a grenade attack on an army lorry he was travelling in. He had been discharged on medical grounds, but despite now having healed physically, he reported difficulties settling back home, as well as frequent nightmares in which he would see friends being killed as well as those people who he had himself killed. In addition to visiting the village health clinic, where he was seen by a medical assistant and Bracken, the former soldier saw a traditional healer. This healer diagnosed him as suffering from the effects of *mayembe* (horned charms), requiring his family to sacrifice a chicken and attend to other rituals. According to Bracken, 'The young man felt relieved when these had been performed and also felt closer to his family'.[106]

We should not assume, however, that community and traditional healers always provided necessary support. In cases of rape, social attitudes, including assumptions about its effects on fertility, made it difficult for many women to talk openly about their experiences.[107] Political considerations and fear also limited the ability of individuals who were otherwise well positioned to offer support, to do so. Teachers, for example, may have been reluctant to show concern for their students because 'their class rooms contained students from different tribal backgrounds whose parents came from a variety of backgrounds—some from the military and others, supporters of the guerrilla movement'. 'Severe reprisals', as Dodge and Raundalen noted, 'were not uncommon for any one who was even suspected to be sympathetic to one side or the other', meaning it was safest to focus on teaching.[108] Cleansing rituals, moreover, did not always offer the unambiguously positive role purported by observers in the Luwero Triangle. Some elders in Acholi and Madi were unwilling to cleanse returning soldiers at ancestral shrines, 'aware that these young men had killed indiscriminately'.[109] The soldiers, moreover, likely 'had no intention of submitting to the authority of elders, or to a ceremony at which they might be publicly castigated for their behaviour'.[110] Alice Lakwena's initiation ceremony, meanwhile, which included placing her hands on the heads of new recruits and cleansing them of past actions, offered a way out of the dilemma of cleansing.[111]

In the context of long histories of war and violence, and in a situation where most were now living in extreme poverty and deprivation, it seems likely that many got by just because they had to. This is perhaps best illustrated by the stories told by street children immediately following the coup in Kampala on 27 July 1985. As one boy recounted:

> On Saturday, 27 July, people were running, and I asked 'Why do you run?'
> Soldiers started to come, running, shooting up in the air and around.
> I thought, the soldiers will enter the market and steal everything. I moved out my bicycle. I started to ride hard. At Queens Way the soldiers were stopping all the cars. I saw a roadblock ahead, many military. They were looting motorcycles, money, watches, everything. I didn't stop. I found a small place where I could pass. They didn't contact me on my bicycle. I rode like a bullet straight home. I found cars breaking down on the way. No number plates. Shooting. When cars fail, people loot tyres, seats, everything.
> Stay home, I told my brothers.
> On Monday, I found dead people on the way. All shops were empty. For me I was just surviving. I was feeling bad because of the shooting. I came back to the market to help white people find food - you know my job.[112]

Such accounts represent anecdotal evidence from children who likely had their own reasons for telling the stories they did to the researchers. But the same can also be said of many other reports of coping, healing and support. Researchers who recorded them had already decided that they were potentially significant forms of knowledge and imbued them with their own assumptions about how individuals and communities were coping.

CONCLUSION

In the context of growing international concern about violence in central Africa during the 1990s, Uganda has occupied an ambiguous space, being relatively peaceful when compared to its neighbours—Democratic Republic of Congo, Rwanda and Sudan. But, in part due to geographical location, being English speaking, and the reputation of Museveni's government for rehabilitation policies, Uganda has also provided a space in which international researchers have felt comfortable, and where humanitarian organisations, looking during the 1990s to move their work beyond the classic emergency response, have been able to expand their ideas about what constitutes a 'crisis', particularly with regard to mental health.[113] Research on depression, anxiety, stress, 'war trauma' and PTSD, conducted in Uganda from the early 1980s, went on to comprise the start of an international body of knowledge about the psychological effects of war and violence in Africa. By the early 2000s, this international body of knowledge and related practices was starting to include psychosocial programmes as essential elements of conflict resolution and peacebuilding. As part of this, leading international humanitarian organisations such as the International Committee of the Red Cross (ICRC) and MSF have prioritised programmes focused on preventing violence and mitigating its effects on health and health care.[114] This recognition of violence as a global public health issue, requiring targeted interventions, has a more complex history than that told here in relation to the psychological effects of war and violence in eastern Africa—it also spans concerns about homicide and gun violence in the USA, the recognition of domestic violence and child abuse in Europe and the USA as social issues, and the rise of epidemiology in contexts around the world, among other themes.[115] Yet Uganda provided a space for the first research into war-related trauma and distress in Africa—one guided by the interests and priorities of international 'experts'.

The fashion for psychosocial programmes in conflict and post-conflict settings has not been without criticism from psychiatrists, humanitarian practitioners, anthropologists and civil society groups. It has been tied to wider critiques of humanitarianism, in which foreign knowledge has been privileged, conflicts depoliticised and historical contexts ignored, and in which legitimacy has been conferred on a certain type of suffering body.[116] Within psychiatry, it has also been influenced by the aims of cross-cultural psychiatry, which has questioned the knowledge-base on which these programmes have been justified.[117] Bracken and Giller, for example, both questioned the idea that trauma existed in a state waiting to be 'found' by an expert, as well as the assumption that those meeting the clinical definition of PTSD would not be able to recover without professional (Western-trained) help.[118] More broadly, critiques of psychosocial programmes have centred on their lack of integration into wider health and medical systems, fatigue amongst those targeted by NGOs for support and the lack of regulation regarding approaches. Voluntary Service Overseas (VSO) reportedly ran a psychosocial programme in Uganda in the mid-1990s, involving counselling, but was 'widely criticised for not being integrated in any sustainable public health structure'.[119] A participant at a UNHRC and WHO-funded Community-Based Rehabilitation Workshop in Kampala in 1996 suggested that one of the main problems of such programmes was 'too many agencies and lack of proper communication channels'.[120] In 2000, moreover, Harrell-Bond reported concerns about well-funded agencies in northern Uganda that were working with former child soldiers of the LRA. 'The "therapies" offered', she noted, 'are diverse. For example, some insist on the religious conversion of these children'.[121] This, among one agency, was regarded 'as more important than reuniting children with their parents...in one case at least the parents were not informed for more than a year that their child was safe'.[122]

As Uganda's psychiatrists remobilised during the 1990s, they became actively involved in projects aimed at providing support to those affected by violence. In the early 1990s, Mungherera established the NGO 'Hope after Rape' for women who had been raped during the insurgency in northern Uganda, to which other psychiatrists also contributed.[123] She highlighted the lack of counselling services in northern Uganda, as well as a broader need to help women.[124] Mungherera also worked as a part-time consultant for the Transcultural Psychosocial Organisation from 1998, ran a mental health service for Sudanese refugees in the Adjumani, Moyo and Arua Districts of northern Uganda and trained psychiatric nurses and counsellors to expand the work.[125] Nakasi, moreover, became a consultant for the African Centre for the Treatment and Rehabilitation of Torture Victims (ACTV), established in Kampala in 1993 to provide rehabilitation services to survivors of torture.[126] She worked there until 1998, when her claim that 90% of female inmates in prisons were raped by prison warders led to her dismissal and indictment.[127] Yet despite this increasing involvement, which since the 2000s has extended to leading research on trauma, Uganda's psychiatrists have remained largely absent in wider critiques of the methods and approaches used in psychosocial programmes. In the context of ongoing struggles to establish authority over mental illness, claims to the universality of concepts of trauma have remained dominant.

NOTES

1. S. R. Karugire, *A Political History of Uganda* (Kampala, 2010), p. 197.
2. H. Dinwiddy, 'The Ugandan Army and Makerere Under Obote, 1962–71', *African Affairs* 82(326) (1983), p. 59.
3. H. B. Hansen, 'Uganda in the 1970s: A Decade of Paradoxes and Ambiguities', *Journal of Eastern African Studies* 7(1) (2013), pp. 87–92.
4. R. Reid, *A History of Modern Uganda* (Cambridge, 2017), p. 60.
5. A. K. Hundle, 'Exceptions to the Expulsion: Violence, Security and Community Among Ugandan Asians, 1972–79', *Journal of Eastern African Studies* 7(1) (2013), pp. 164–182.
6. Reid, *A History of Modern Uganda*, p. 61.
7. G. Roberts, 'The Uganda–Tanzania War, the Fall of Idi Amin, and the Failure of African Diplomacy, 1978–1979', *Journal of Eastern African Studies* 8(4) (2014), pp. 692–709.
8. Reid, *A History of Modern Uganda*, pp. 71–76.
9. Ibid., p. 75.
10. P. J. Bracken, J. E. Giller, and S. Kabaganda, 'Helping Victims of Violence in Uganda', *Medicine and War* 8(3) (1992), p. 159.
11. *The Report of the Commission of Inquiry into Violations of Human Rights: Verbatim Record of Proceedings*, vol. 1 (Kampala, 1994), pp. 348–366.
12. D. M. Anderson and Ø. H. Rolandsen, 'Violence as Politics in Eastern Africa, 1940–1990: Legacy, Agency, Contingency', *Journal of Eastern African Studies* 8(4) (2014), p. 543. See also, A. B. K. Kasozi, *The Social Origins of Violence in Uganda, 1964–1985* (Montreal, 1994), pp. 4–5.
13. R. Doom and K. Vlassenroot, 'Kony's Message: A New *Koine*? The Lord's Resistance Army in Northern Uganda', *African Affairs* 98(390) (1999), pp. 5–36. On Alice Lakwena, see especially T. Allen, 'Understanding Alice: Uganda's Holy Spirit Movement in Context', *Africa: Journal of the International African Institute* 61(3) (1991), pp. 370–399; and H. Behrend, *Alice Lakwena and the Holy Spirits: War in Northern Uganda, 1985–97* (Ohio, 2000).
14. See especially, A. Branch, *Displacing Human Rights: War and Intervention in Northern Uganda* (Oxford, 2011).

15. J. Kibuka-Musoke, 'Amin's Madness by His Doctor: Exclusive', *The Observer*, 1 May 1977, p. 11.
16. C. Lamwaka, 'Civil War and the Peace Process in Uganda, 1986–1997', *East African Journal of Peace and Human Rights* 4(2) (1998), p. 160.
17. See, for example, 'The Deadly Cult of Joseph Kony', *The Independent*, 8 November 2000; 'A Psychiatrist's Take on LRA Leader Kony', *New Vision*, 1 June 2006.
18. J. Bevan, 'The Myth of Madness: Cold Rationality and 'Resource' Plunder by the Lord's Resistance Army', *Civil Wars* 9(4) (2007), pp. 343–358. See also, T. Allen and K. Vlassenroot, eds., *The Lord's Resistance Army: Myth and Reality* (London, 2010); M. Leopold, *Inside West Nile: Violence, History and Representation on an African Frontier* (Oxford, 2005); and R. Vokes, *Ghosts of Kanungu: Fertility, Secrecy & Exchange in the Great Lakes of East Africa* (Kampala, 2009).
19. Reid, *A History of Modern Uganda*, p. 63. See also, D. M. Anderson, 'Exit from Empire: Counter-Insurgency and Decolonization in Kenya, 1952–1963,' in T. Clack and R. Johnson, eds., *At the End of Military Intervention: Historical, Theoretical and Applied Solutions to Transition, Handover and Withdrawal* (Oxford, 2014).
20. See D. Fassin and R. Rechtman, *The Empire of Trauma: An Inquiry into the Condition of Victimhood* (Princeton, 2009).
21. B. Harrell-Bond, 'Foreword', in F. L. Ahearn, ed., *Psychosocial Wellness of Refugees: Issues in Qualitative and Quantitative Research* (New York, 2000), p. xii.
22. World Health Organization, *Prevention of Violence: A Public Health Priority*, Forty-Ninth World Health Assembly Resolution (Geneva, 20 May 1996).
23. As cited in Branch, *Displacing Human Rights*, pp. 135–136.
24. J. E. Walugembe (Post-humus), 'A Pioneer's Look at Psychotrauma in Uganda "Post-traumatic Stress Disorder as Seen in Mulago Hospital Mental Health Clinic (1992)"', *African Journal of Traumatic Stress* 1(1) (2010), pp. 6–18.
25. *The Report of the Commission of Inquiry into Violations of Human Rights: Verbatim Record of Proceedings*, vol. 4 (Kampala 1994), pp. 3834–3910.
26. J. Iliffe, *East African Doctors: A History of the Modern Profession* (Kampala, 2002), p. 146.
27. Uganda Ministry of Health Archives (UMOHA) PH/HP/8 (Box 30 New) (Butabika Hospital), f. 111, 'Butabika Hospital: A Case for Rehabilitation', 25 January 1993, p. 1; Uganda Ministry of Health Library (UMOHL), Raphael Owor, 'Report and Recommendations of the Health Policy Review Commission' (Unpublished report, 1987), pp. 72–73.

28. World Health Organization Library (WHOL) MNH/POL/87.3, *African Mental Health Action Group, Tenth Meeting* (Geneva, 1987), p. 9.
29. Albert Cook Memorial Library, Makerere University (ACMM), G. G. C. Rwegellera, 'The Present State of Mental Health Services in Uganda and Proposals for Their Re-organization, 1985–1986', Unpublished paper, p. 11.
30. Personal communication with G. A. German, 29 January 2012.
31. Personal communication with German.
32. Personal communication with German.
33. World Health Organization Archives (WHOA) M-PROJECTS UGANDA HMD-001 (Faculty of Medicine, Makerere University, Uganda), f. 3, 'First Semi-Annual Project Report 1st October–30th November 1975'; Personal communication with W. Acuda, 21 October 2011.
34. UMOHA C90/ACR (Bosa Stephen B—Consult. Psychiat.), f. 134, letter from S. B. Bosa, to the Permanent Secretary for Establishments, Entebbe, 31 May 1972; UMOHA C90/ACR, f. 138, letter from S. L. N. Serwanja, for Permanent Secretary for Establishments, to the Permanent Secretary, Ministry of Health, 28 March 1973; and UMOHA C90/ACR, f. 139, letter from J. K. Barugahara, Ministry of Health, to the Secretary, Public Service Commission, 31 January 1973.
35. Jinja District Archives (JDA) Med 4/1 (Psychiatric).
36. JDA Med 4/1, 'Minutes of the Busoga Psychiatric Advisory Committee Meeting Held on 14th November, 1973 in the Library of Jinja Hospital at 4.00 p.m.', p. 3.
37. See, for example, UMOHA PH/HP/8 (Butabika Hospital), f. 63, letter from A. M. Kitumba to the Provincial Engineer, Kampala, 25 November 1977.
38. Personal communication with J. Bossa, 6 July 2012; H. G. Egdell, 'Obituary of Steven Bosa', *The Psychiatrist* 25 (2001).
39. Personal communication with Bossa.
40. UMOHA C90/ACR, f. 146, letter from Ben Kawooya, Medical Superintendent, to The Director of Medical Services, Entebbe, 14 November 1988.
41. UMOHA PHC/HP/2 (Hospital—Butabika Hospital), f. 25, letter from Ben Kawooya to the Hon. Minister of Health, Entebbe, 13 May 1988, p. 3.
42. UMOHA PHC/HP/2, f. 25, letter from Ben Kawooya to the Hon. Minister of Health, Entebbe, 13 May 1988, p. 3; WHOL MNH/POL/88.2, 'Mental Health Leadership Training Workshop, Arusha, Tanzania, 3–14 August 1987', p. 19.

43. Interview with Sheila Ndyanabangi (NDY-01), Ministry of Health, Kampala, 3 May 2011.
44. F. Baingana, 'Use Made of Ward 16 Old Mulago and Butabika Hospital: Patients Views About the Traditional Healer' (Unpublished MMed dissertation, Makerere University, 1987).
45. A. Green, 'Margaret Mungherera', *The Lancet* 389 (March 2017), p. 1188.
46. UMOHA PHC/HP/2, f. 25, letter from Ben Kawooya to the Hon. Minister of Health, Entebbe, 13 May 1988, p. 2.
47. UMOHA PHC/HP/2, f. 23, Ben Kawooya, 'Speech of the Medical Superintendent on the Occasion of the Visit of The Prime Minister Right Honourable Dr. Samson Kiseka Prime Minister of Uganda', September 1987, p. 2.
48. Ibid., p. 2.
49. Ibid., p. 1.
50. Ibid., pp. 1–2.
51. UMOHA PHC/HP/2, f. 33, Sam Barasa, 'Management and Administration of Butabika Hospital—Report (1991–1994)', 3 October 1994.
52. B. E. Harrell-Bond, *Imposing Aid: Emergency Assistance to Refugees* (Oxford, 1986), p. xiii.
53. Harrell-Bond, 'Foreword', p. xii.
54. Harrell-Bond, *Imposing Aid*, p. 323.
55. Ibid., pp. 292–293.
56. Ibid., p. 323.
57. Ibid., pp. 303–304.
58. Ibid., p. 304.
59. Ibid., p. 305.
60. Ibid., p. 283.
61. Ibid., p. 286.
62. See J. Orley and J. K. Wing, 'Psychiatric Disorders in Two African Villages', *Archives of General Psychiatry* 36(5) (1979), pp. 513–520.
63. Harrell-Bond, *Imposing Aid*, pp. 287–288.
64. Ibid., p. 288.
65. See Orley and Wing, 'Psychiatric Disorders in Two African Villages', p. 517.
66. M. Raundalen et al., 'Four Investigations on Stress among Children in Uganda', in C. P. Dodge and M. Raundalen, eds., *War, Violence and Children in Uganda* (Oslo, 1987), p. 84.
67. A. Dyregrov and M. Raundalen, 'Children and the Stresses of War—A Review', in Dodge and Raundalen, eds., *War, Violence and Children in Uganda*, p. 111.

68. C. P. Dodge and M. Raundalen, *Reaching Children in War: Sudan, Uganda and Mozambique* (Bergen, 1991); Raundalen et al., 'Four Investigations on Stress', p. 84.
69. Raundalen et al., 'Four Investigations on Stress', p. 100.
70. Ibid.
71. Ibid.
72. Dodge and Raundalen, *Reaching Children in War*, p. 90.
73. E. Hooper and L. Pirouet, *Uganda*, The Minority Rights Group Report No. 66 (1989), p. 20.
74. L. Weisæth, 'Torture of a Norwegian Ship's Crew: The Torture, Stress Reactions and Psychiatric After-Effects', *Acta Psychiatrica Scandinavica* 80(s355) (1989), pp. 63–72; F. E. Somnier and I. K. Genefke, 'Psychotherapy for Victims of Torture', *The British Journal of Psychiatry* 149(3) (1986), pp. 323–329.
75. J. Giller, 'Caring for "Victims of Torture" in Uganda: Some Personal Reflections', in P. J. Bracken and C. Petty, eds., *Rethinking the Trauma of War* (London, 1998), p. 128.
76. Hooper and Pirouet, *Uganda*, p. 24.
77. Ibid., p. 131.
78. Ibid., p. 132.
79. Ibid., p. 133.
80. Ibid., p. 142.
81. Bracken, Giller, and Kabaganda, 'Helping Victims of Violence', pp. 158–159.
82. Bracken, Giller, and Kabaganda, 'Helping Victims of Violence'.
83. P. J. Bracken, J. E. Giller, and D. Summerfield, 'Rethinking Mental Health Work with Survivors of Wartime Violence and Refugees', *Journal of Refugee Studies* 10(4) (1997), pp. 431–442; P. J. Bracken, J. E. Giller, and D. Summerfield, 'Psychological Responses to War and Atrocity: The Limitations of Current Concepts', *Social Science & Medicine* 40(8) (1995), pp. 1073–1082.
84. P. Redfield, 'The Verge of Crisis: Doctors Without Borders in Uganda', in D. Fassin and M. Pandolfi, eds., *Contemporary States of Emergency: The Politics of Military and Humanitarian Interventions* (New York, 2010). On violence in central Africa in the 1990s, see especially G. Prunier, *Africa's World War: Congo, the Rwandan Genocide, and the Making of a Continental Catastrophe* (Oxford, 2009).
85. Bertrand Taithe has highlighted similar use of Cambodian refugee camps in 'The Cradle of the New Humanitarian System? International Work and European Volunteers at the Cambodian Border Camps, 1979–1993', *Contemporary European History* 25(2) (May 2016), pp. 335–358.

86. A. Branch, 'Humanitarianism, Violence, and the Camp in Northern Uganda', *Civil Wars* 11(4) (2009), pp. 477–501; L. N. Moro, 'Interethnic Relations in Exile: The Politics of Ethnicity Among Sudanese Refugees in Uganda and Egypt', *Journal of Refugee Studies* 17(4) (2004), pp. 420–436.

87. WHOA M4-372-28 (Collaboration between WHO & IPSER regarding the International Programme on the Psychosocial Consequences of War among Refugees & Displaced Persons), 'Netherlands/WHO Annual Review Meeting, Geneva, 5–6 December 1991'.

88. WHOA M4-372-28, J. de Jong, 'Project Proposal for an Intervention Project on the Identification, Management and Prevention of Psycho-Social and Mental Health Problems of Refugees and other Victims of Man-Made Disaster in Northern Uganda', February 1996, p. 3.

89. WHOA M4-372-28, de Jong, 'Project Proposal for an Intervention Project', p. 6.

90. WHOA M4-372-28, de Jong, 'Project Proposal for an Intervention Project', pp. 6–7.

91. J. T. V. M. de Jong, 'Prevention of the Consequences of Man-Made or Natural Disaster at the (Inter)National, the Community, the Family and the Individual Level', in S. E. Hobfoll and M. W. de Vries, eds., *Extreme Stress and Communities: Impact and Intervention* (Dordrecht, 1995), p. 207.

92. Walugembe, 'A Pioneer's Look at Psychotrauma', pp. 6–18.

93. A. Brett, 'Testimonies of War Trauma in Uganda', in T. Allen, ed., *In Search of Cool Ground: War, Flight and Homecoming in Northeast Africa* (Laurenceville, 1996), p. 278.

94. Giller, 'Caring for "Victims of Torture"', p. 134.

95. Giller, 'Caring for "Victims of Torture"', p. 143.

96. Harrell-Bond, *Imposing Aid*, p. 319.

97. P. J. Bracken, 'Trauma and the Age of Postmodernity: A Hermeneutic Approach to Post Traumatic Anxiety' (Unpublished PhD thesis, University of Warwick, 1998), p. 124.

98. Bracken, 'Trauma and the Age of Postmodernity', p. 123.

99. Dodge and Raundalen, *Reaching Children in War*, p. 109.

100. Bracken, 'Trauma and the Age of Postmodernity', pp. 120–121.

101. Dodge and Raundalen, *Reaching Children in War*, p. 110.

102. WHOA M4-372-28, de Jong, 'Project Proposal for an Intervention Project', p. 8.

103. Ibid.

104. Ibid.

105. Walugembe, 'A Pioneer's Look at Psychotrauma', pp. 13–14.

106. Bracken, 'Trauma and the Age of Postmodernity', pp. 124–125.

107. Giller, 'Caring for "Victims of Torture"'.
108. Dodge and Raundalen, *Reaching Children in War*, p. 107.
109. Allen, 'Understanding Alice', p. 378.
110. Ibid.
111. Ibid. See also Behrend, *Alice Lakwena and the Holy Spirits*, p. 49.
112. A. Dyregrov and M. Raundalen, 'Children and the Stresses of War—A Review', in Dodge and Raundalen, eds., *War, Violence and Children in Uganda*, p. 127.
113. Redfield, 'The Verge of Crisis', p. 177.
114. V. Bernard, 'Violence Against Health Care: Giving in Is Not an Option', *International Review of the Red Cross* 95(889) (2013), pp. 5–12; M. Le Pape and P. Salignon, eds., *Civilians Under Fire: Humanitarian Practices in the Congo Republic 1998–2000* (Brussels, 2003); and M. Ticktin, 'The Gendered Human of Humanitarianism: Medicalising and Politicising Sexual Violence', *Gender & History* 23(2) (2011), pp. 250–265.
115. L. L. Dahlberg and J. A. Mercy, 'History of Violence as a Public Health Problem', *Virtual Mentor: American Medical Association Journal of Ethics* 11(2) (2009), pp. 167–172.
116. S. Abramowitz and C. Panter-Brick, 'Bringing Life into Relief: Comparative Ethnographies of Humanitarian Practice', in S. Abramowitz and C. Panter-Brick, eds., *Medical Humanitarianism: Ethnographies of Practice* (Philadelphia, 2015); Fassin and Rechtman, *The Empire of Trauma*; and L. H. Malkki, 'Speechless Emissaries: Refugees, Humanitarianism, and Dehistoricization', *Cultural Anthropology* 11(3) (1996), pp. 377–404.
117. D. Summerfield, 'A Critique of Seven Assumptions Behind Psychological Trauma Programmes in War-Affected Areas', *Social Science & Medicine* 48(10) (1999), pp. 1449–1462.
118. Bracken, Giller, and Summerfield, 'Rethinking Mental Health Work', pp. 431–442.
119. WHOA M4-372-28, letter from J. T. V. M. de Jong to Mr. Faubert, UNHRC Nairobi, 8 November 1993, p. 3.
120. WHOL NAD/UNHCR/WHO/RHB.9, *Equal Opportunities for All: A Community-Based Rehabilitation Project for Refugees, Kampala, Uganda, 23–27 September 1996*, p. 1.
121. Harrell-Bond, 'Foreword', p. xiii.
122. Harrell-Bond, 'Foreword', p. xiv.
123. J. Boardman and E. Ovuga, 'Rebuilding Psychiatry in Uganda', *Psychiatric Bulletin* 21(10) (1997), p. 651; Green, 'Margaret Mungherera', p. 1188.
124. Green, 'Margaret Mungherera', p. 1188.

125. 'Dr Margaret Mungherera: Influence Beyond Borders', *Daily Monitor*, 27 October 2012.
126. B. Githiora, 'The African Centre for the Treatment and Rehabilitation of Torture Victims: Treating the Terrified', *Executive*, December 1993, pp. 43–44.
127. N. L. Wamboka, 'Uganda: Dr Nakasi's Sacking Is Bad for Women In-Mates', *The Monitor*, 9 June 1998.

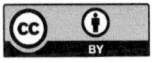

CHAPTER 8

Conclusion

At a World Health Organization (WHO) meeting in 2012, Robinah Alambuya, Information Officer at the NGO Mental Health Uganda and Chair of the Pan African Network of People with Psychosocial Disabilities (PANUSP), declared that:

> The history of psychiatry haunts our present. Our people remain chained and shackled in institutions and by ideas which colonisers brought to our continent and many other parts of the world. Indeed, we do remain 'objects of treatment and charity' and some of the worst human rights violations do occur in the very institutions that claim to provide mental health care services.[1]

Alambuya, who has lived with bipolar disorder for over twenty years, is one of the most passionate members of the mental health service user movement in Uganda. Although she has had many negative experiences in navigating the psychiatric system, she does not believe that psychiatry is incapable of offering relief to those suffering from mental illness. Rather, she cannot see why psychiatric services and disability legislation have failed to evolve to meet the needs of those they claim to help and protect. Parliamentary discussions over the reform of the Mental Health Treatment Act exemplify this lack of change. First enacted under colonial rule and last revised in 1964, the Act does not differentiate between different types of mental disorder, largely neglects community care,

© The Author(s) 2019
Y. Pringle, *Psychiatry and Decolonisation in Uganda,*
Mental Health in Historical Perspective,
https://doi.org/10.1057/978-1-137-60095-0_8

and defines those with mental health disabilities as 'persons of unsound mind' and 'idiots'.[2] Such is the power of its outdated and derogatory language that the law is regarded as one that 'spurs more injustice than justice'.[3] Alambuya, for one, maintains that it has led to the exclusion of mental health service users from the processes of reform. Yet:

> There can be no mental health without embracing our expertise. We have always remained the untapped resource in mental health care. We must be involved and consulted in raising awareness, service delivery, monitoring and finding solutions to the barriers faced by users and survivors of psychiatry and people with psychosocial disabilities.[4]

When history is evoked in discussions like these, it is often done to stress the perceived failings, even irrelevance, of psychiatry. Commentators draw attention to divergences between 'modern' or 'international' psychiatric practices and those in Uganda; they focus on outdated mental health legislation and psychiatric facilities, all of them relics of the colonial period. In a successful petition to the Constitutional Court in 2011, human rights lawyers at the Centre for Health, Human Rights and Development (CEHURD) and Daniel Iga, a mental health service user, contested degrading practices and use of language towards people with mental disabilities in the criminal justice system. They argued that individuals who had been acquitted of a crime by reason of insanity should not be kept in custody indefinitely, because this contravened 'the right to liberty and freedom from discrimination' guaranteed by the Constitution. They also challenged the use of the words 'idiot' and 'imbecile' in the Penal Code Act—language that had not been changed since 1950—and argued that the word 'lunatic' was dehumanising and devoid of any form of dignity. In doing so, they set colonial attitudes towards mental illness against the hopes and aims of those who had written the 1995 Constitution of Uganda, as well as the Universal Declaration of Human Rights, the International Covenant on Civil and Political Rights, the United Nations Convention on the Rights of Persons with Disabilities (UNCRPD) and the African Charter on Human and Peoples' Rights.[5]

The history of psychiatry and decolonisation reveals a more dynamic picture, with psychiatrists and others actively engaged in processes of innovation and reform, but which, as evidenced by complaints about the unchanging nature of psychiatry, have not had a long-lasting effect within Uganda. This in part reflects the long-contested nature of psychiatric practices, which have always been subject to criticism by those who have navigated them. But it also highlights how psychiatry has been tied to shifting periods of stability, upheaval and crisis. Efforts to reorganise mental health care, and to refigure the relationship between psychiatry and patients, stalled with the political and economic insecurity of the 1970s and 1980s. In the post-conflict context, it has proved difficult to revitalise psychiatry, with government policies only adding to the perception of psychiatry as static and unchanging. Like other areas of medicine and health, the government's approach to the rebuilding of services during the 1980s and 1990s prioritised the physical rehabilitation of existing infrastructure, failing to use the opportunity to rethink the organisation of services and ignoring, as Joanna Macrae, Anthony Zwi and Lucy Gilson have noted, 'issues of equity and sustainability'.[6] Despite the dominance of decentralised approaches and the policy of mental health in primary care within international mental health, psychiatric services remained highly centralised, with Butabika Hospital as the focal point of psychiatric provision and expertise. While mental health was included in the First Health Policy of the National Policy and Health Sector Strategic Plan in 1999, moves towards integrating mental health in primary care were not made until the early 2000s.[7]

During the 1990s and 2000s, psychiatry was actively promoted within Makerere Medical School, first under the leadership of Emilio Ovuga and then under Seggane Musisi. Yet change has nevertheless been slow, with psychiatry and mental health remaining one of the most neglected areas of medicine. As of October 2017, there were 33 registered psychiatrists to serve a population of approximately 38 million, over half of whom were based in or on the outskirts of Kampala.[8] Approximately 1% of the government's national health care expenditure is directed towards mental health, and this seems unlikely to change in the near future. Of this, just over half is directed towards Butabika.[9] Patients who are admitted to Butabika receive food and have free access to essential psychotropic medicines, but because of severe shortages of personnel, patients tend to be heavily medicated. Outpatient care is growing but can be expensive. A WHO survey in 2006 found that approximately 37% of the daily minimum wage was needed to pay for one day's worth of antipsychotic medication while approximately 7% of the daily wage was needed to pay for one dose of antidepressants.[10]

Many of the challenges facing psychiatrists today are reminiscent of those experienced by psychiatrists as they took over responsibility for psychiatry at the end of empire—those of underdevelopment, financial neglect, large custodial institutions and low prestige. In the contexts of development and nation building, and facing ongoing difficulties in persuading government officials of the importance of psychiatry, psychiatrists challenged their prescribed custodial and curative roles. They took on social advisory roles and experimented with new ways of delivering mental health care. While patients were not given a voice, their activities were premised not only on the assumption that demand on psychiatry would only grow in the future, but that action needed to be taken to bring psychiatry closer to the mentally ill. Nor was psychiatry limited to the national context during the years of decolonisation. While local and national political and economic forces shaped the ability of psychiatrists to participate in international mental health, during the 1960s and early 1970s, Uganda became a prominent voice in regional and international discussions on the organisation of mental health services in developing countries. While there was a broad divide within Africa between English- and French-speaking nations, psychiatrists found common ground in a sense of shared challenges in their professional lives. The practical experiences of psychiatrists in experimenting with mental health care during the 1960s and 1970s came to dominate international discussions on mental health care, feeding into the WHO's policy on mental health in primary care.

Today, most Ugandans are aware of the existence and purpose of Butabika Hospital, whether through word of mouth or informative articles published in newspapers like the *Daily Monitor* or the *New Vision*. Yet it is clear that psychiatry, perhaps more than any other medical discipline, has lingered on the edge of a much broader therapeutic landscape. In a study of severe mental illness in two districts in eastern Uganda, Catherine Abbo reported that just as communities drew on multiple explanatory models for psychosis, they also sought multiple solutions. 'Traditional healing and biomedical services', she noted, 'were used concurrently by over 80% of the subjects'.[11] Uganda is not unique here. In a study of the routes to psychiatric care centres in Nigeria, Oye Gureje and colleagues found that spiritual healers, traditional healers and general practitioners were the first to be consulted by 13, 19, and 47% of patients, respectively.[12] Explanations of why psychiatry has been and remains a last resort for so many necessarily touch on questions of cost, distance and the perceived severity of symptoms. But they also reveal much about differing ways of understanding, communicating and treating mental illness, as well as the difficulties psychiatry has had as a discipline in claiming universal models for understanding the mind. While concerns about the social and cultural gap between psychiatrists and their patients occupied a central position in justifying the Africanisation of psychiatry, as well as in arguments for reform during the years of decolonisation, the gulf between psychiatrists and patients was not resolved.

Despite the ongoing challenges facing psychiatry, the mental health landscape in Uganda today has never been more vibrant. Since 2010, there has been a proliferation of mental health organisations, increasingly led by people with lived experience of mental illness, and which are engaged in outreach activities and home visits in urban communities. An increasing number of organisations are also working to build capacity in mental health activism and self-advocacy, drawing on the skills and knowledge of service users, as well as sympathetic allies such as journalists and occupational therapists. In the absence of a large body of Ugandan psychiatrists, and in the context of low government investment in mental health, the global mental health movement has entered the psychiatric landscape, creating new alliances and shaping perceptions of rights and how to claim them. One of these alliances is an international health partnership between Butabika and the East London NHS Foundation Trust, set up in 2005, and known as the Butabika-East London Link. They have worked with mental health service users to bid for funding, facilitated international exchanges and are currently among those working with peer support workers at Butabika Hospital to provide recovery-oriented training and support in a new Recovery College.[13] Such alliances are connecting a select group of Ugandans to global bodies of knowledge and ways of talking about mental illness in ways that evoke the wider literature on 'global citizenship' in medicine and health.[14] As such, the nascent mental health movement raises important questions about the politics of intermediaries, knowledge and legitimacy, as well as who is included and who is left out. Terminology is also difficult, as the use of the terms 'service users' and 'survivors' risk excluding the vast majority of those in Uganda who suffer from mental illness but who either do not have access to western medical services or who choose to seek different forms of therapy. Many of those involved in mental health organisations are aware of these problems of terminology, and as such, a wide variety of terms are in use, including 'people with lived experience of mental illness', 'people with psychosocial disabilities', and 'people with mental health problems'.[15] In spite of this, there is still slippage and conflation of these terms.

Mental health organisations started to proliferate in the mid-1990s in the context of what has been referred to as 'the NGO-isation of society'.[16] In 1999, Mental Health Uganda was founded. Mainly donor-funded, it came to operate across 18 districts, setting up drug banks to ensure the consistency of medication supply and organising group saving schemes, with provision for start-up loans so members might have an opportunity to generate income and contribute to their families' well-being. Other organisations included the Uganda Schizophrenia Fellowship, with active user bases in Masaka and Jinja, and Basic Needs Uganda, which remains a leader in advocacy training and income generation projects across the country. The organisation which pioneered service user involvement, however, was Heartsounds. Founded in 2008 in collaboration with mental health service users and psychiatrists in the Butabika-East London Link, Heartsounds defined itself as being the first to truly tap what it referred to as the under-utilised resource of people with lived experience of mental illness. It was the first organisation to be run entirely by service users, aiming to create a community in which people could share their stories about treatment, the problems encountered in daily life, and build a sense of belonging among members. According to one founder member, 'When one peer visits another and talks they give hope. If this one can do it then the other one can do it'. Led by Joseph Atukunda, the organisation had a base in Kampala, with its own Internet café, library and guest house. By 2013, it had 107 registered members, including service users, 'survivors' and mental health professionals. Until 2016, when the organisation disbanded, it had a board of trustees which comprised of seven mental health service users (including Alambuya), a caretaker and three advisory members who were leaders of other mental health organisations.

Heartsounds were vocal about the importance of speaking out about mental illness and giving testimony as a way of fighting stigma and discrimination. This was particularly important because many of the more prominent members of Heartsounds were relatively well-educated and from financially stable backgrounds—not the stereotypical mad person seen wandering the streets in rags. They created a website containing film clips of members giving testimony about their lives and journeys to recovery. These testimonies fell into remarkably similar patterns, centred around periods of 'crisis' from which they are now in recovery. It was clear that there were many stories of discrimination, prejudice and stigma, but also messages that suffering could be overcome. Much of the language used reflected the international and even global outlook of organisations such as these, particularly in their use of terms such as 'crisis' and 'recovery', and in statements about patient rights. One of the videos showed Daniel, a teacher who for a long time did not want to be open about his mental health problems for fear of what his students might think. He explained, 'When I was young I used to see *mulalu* (a mad person) and I was like, what did they do? You know perhaps people have say here don't mind him he robbed someone so they bewitched him. I know that mystery, but the end of the day he's a human being, whose mind is a bit disoriented, and he needs to be taken care of'. Another video showed Elizabeth, who had a history of alcohol and drug abuse, and had suffered from depression for a few years. In her words, 'It was at Heartsounds that I first found comments of, "wow, you're brilliant", "wow, you can do this". Those comments first came from Heartsounds'. Elizabeth continued to explain how with family you could do good things and you could do bad, but 'they are always ready to criticise the bad...And you can live life knowing you can never do anything good'.[17]

For the first few years, the peer support work pioneered by Heartsounds was relatively informal, but in 2012, the Butabika-East London Link was successful in securing funding from DfID and the Tropical Health and Education Trust to run 'Brain Gain'. This project formalised and expanded peer support work by training approximately thirty-six peer support workers over a two-year period. Peer supporters then went out into communities in Kampala and met with people who had recently been released from Butabika.[18] While the project reportedly had success in convincing psychiatrists at Butabika, who had initially been resistant, of the benefits of the approach, overall the project faced financial mismanagement and fraud, with some of the money from the international partnership being diverted into other projects. Some of those involved also point to power struggles within Heartsounds, with some feeling that Atukunda was not mentally stable enough to run the organisation, and that women who had childcare commitments were being pushed out of peer support work. When the Butabika-East London Link was successful in securing funding for 'Brain Gain 2' in 2015, the project was moved into Butabika itself. Atukunda was no longer involved, and many of the other original members went on to set up new mental health organisations in and around Kampala. Brain Gain 2 saw the creation of Africa's first Mental Health Recovery College, extending peer support into the wards of Butabika, and providing a centre within the grounds to which patients could come, use the internet, and take part in recovery-oriented training and education. In a project organised by the London School of Hygiene and Tropical Medicine (LSHTM) in 2015–2016, moreover, peer support workers and psychologists worked alongside each other to evaluate peer support and recovery, looking through patient files and identifying 'revolving door' patients in need of special attention.

The movement of peer support into Butabika is just one way in which traditional spaces of psychiatry are being renegotiated by mental health organisations and the global health movement that fund and support them. And this belies any overly simplistic claims of neo-colonialism or cultural imperialism within psychiatry. Peer support workers are reshaping hierarchies at Butabika that have long been rigid and well defined. Since the inception of the Recovery College in 2015, peer support workers have entered the hospital every day, walking freely around the grounds, stopping to greet nurses and requesting appointments with the Executive Director. Although they have not received salaries, they have been sworn in as official officers of Butabika and wear a uniform. This makes the 'peer' aspect of their roles problematic, raising new questions about the roles of peer support workers as intermediaries in psychiatry. It has not been unusual, for example, for a female patient to kneel in front of a male peer support worker when meeting them in the corridor. While this is a normal sign of respect in Uganda, particularly by women, it is suggestive of some of the ways in which peer support workers have become another group of workers within Butabika's hierarchy, occupying a difficult position between patient and staff. Being conversant both in the local languages and in an international language of self-care, they are also in positions to translate information about patient rights and medication. While the peer support workers are clear that medication is a vital part of recovery, and that people should encourage and remind each other to continue with their medication after being discharged from hospital, some of them have doubts and are in positions to share their experiences of adjusting their dosage and negotiating treatment regimes with medical professionals. They talk about how shocked patients are to discover that they do not have to accept all treatments that are offered, that they can question them, and work with their doctors to draw up their own plans. While patients have long contested and challenged psychiatric practices, as seen in this book, the public manner in which patients are encouraged to speak out now sets this work apart.

It is clear that peer support workers have come to occupy an uneasy space at Butabika, something not helped by the reliance on international funding. There have also been concerns about the increasingly close links between mental health services users and psychiatrists, with disagreement as to whether peer support workers are best off working within the system or outside it. As one peer support worker noted, 'as we research more about mental health on the internet by reading books, we have come across some antipsychiatry stuff that we find difficult to ignore'. They referred to the book *Anatomy of an Epidemic* by the American journalist Robert Whitaker, which sees psychiatrists as colluding with the psychopharmaceutical industry in creating an epidemic of mental illness. 'Voicing out our thoughts', they added, 'after reading such stuff, is putting us at loggerheads with the service providers who are meant to be our partners'. Kabale Benon, moreover, was actively involved in court cases against Butabika management while working as a peer support worker in the Recovery College. In 2016, with support from CEHURD, Benon successfully lodged a civil complaint against the Attorney General for mistreatment at Butabika Hospital during two periods of admission, in 2005 and in 2010. While at Butabika, Benon was undressed and locked in seclusion—a small cold dark room measuring about two square metres, and that supposedly helps 'cool' the patient when they are agitated. The room had no windows or source of light, bedding, toilet or urinal. He was forced to urinate and defecate on the floor, sleep on a concrete platform and received no medical attention during this time. The case highlighted how seclusion practices violated the human rights of patients at Butabika Hospital, and were in contravention both of Uganda's Constitution and numerous international conventions on disability rights. Benon won the case in November 2016, received compensation, and, in addition to his peer support work, continued to work to assist with other court cases against Butabika.[19] Increasing antagonism between Benon and the authorities at Butabika, however, saw him removed from the Recovery College in 2018.[20]

The most problematic aspect of the new mental health landscape is the ongoing reliance on international funding. This has shaped aims and goals as well as meaning that many organisations and their projects have been short-lived. In this context, some have started to question the usefulness of the dominant global language of 'scaling up' in mental health care in the Ugandan context. If they had full control, as one staff member at Butabika commented informally, they would prefer instead to 'scale down'—to focus on the most troubled people and really make a difference in their lives. Yet, in spite of such challenges and concerns, many of those involved in Uganda's nascent mental health movement are hopeful about the future and the possibilities for the greater participation of people with mental illness in public life.

NOTES

1. R. Alambuya, 'Human Rights Violations Experienced by People with Psychosocial Disabilities', Keynote address delivered at the Launch of the WHO QualityRights Project and Tool Kit, New York, 28 June 2012.
2. Uganda Government, *The Mental Treatment Act*, Chapter 270, Revised Edition, 1964.
3. C. Nyombi, 'A Critical Review of the Uganda Mental Health Treatment Bill, 2011', *East African Journal of Peace and Human Rights* 18(2) (2012), pp. 499–513.
4. Alambuya, 'Human Rights Violations'.
5. The Counsel for the State did not dispute the petition and the terms 'idiots' and 'imbeciles' have now been removed from the Penal Code. *Uganda Constitutional Petition no. 64 of 2011.*
6. J. MacRae, A. B. Zwi, and L. Gilson, 'A Triple Burden for Health Sector Reform: "Post"-conflict Rehabilitation in Uganda', *Social Science and Medicine* 42(7) (1996), p. 1106.
7. F. Kigozi et al., 'An Overview of Uganda's Mental Health Care System: Results from an Assessment Using the World Health Organization's Assessment Instrument for Mental Health Systems (WHO-AIMS)', *International Journal of Mental Health Systems* 4(1) (2010), p. 2; F. Kigozi and J. Ssebunnya, 'Integration of Mental Health into Primary Health Care in Uganda: Opportunities and Challenges', *Mental Health in Family Medicine* 6 (2009), pp. 37–42; E. Ovuga, J. Boardman, and D. Wasserman, 'Integrating Mental Health into Primary Health Care: Local Initiatives from Uganda', *World Psychiatry* 6(1) (2007), pp. 60–61.
8. Uganda Medical and Dental Practitioners Council, Specialist Register. Available at: www.umdpc.com/registers/Specialist%20Register.xls, last accessed 17 December 2017.
9. Kigozi et al., 'An Overview of Uganda's Mental Health Care System', p. 3.
10. World Health Organization, *WHO proMIND: Profiles on Mental Health in Development: Uganda* (Geneva, 2012), p. 40.

11. C. Abbo, 'Profiles and Outcome of Traditional Healing Practices of Severe Mental Illnesses in Two Districts of Eastern Uganda', *Global Health Action* 4 (2011), p. 11.
12. O. Gureje et al., 'Results from the Ibadan Centre', in T. B. Üstün and N. Sartorius, eds., *Mental Illness in General Health Care: An International Study* (Chichester, 1995), p. 158.
13. D. Baillie et al., 'Diaspora and Peer Support Working: Benefits of and Challenges for the Butabika-East London Link', *BJPsych International* 12(1) (2015), pp. 10–13.
14. See, for example, V.-K. Nguyen, *The Republic of Therapy: Triage and Sovereignty in West Africa's Time of AIDS* (Durham, 2010).
15. This and the following paragraphs are based in part on a series of interviews conducted with peer support workers in Kampala in August and September 2016. The interviewees are listed in the bibliography, but I have not attributed statements here in order to protect their privacy.
16. J. Hearn, 'The "NGO-Isation" of Kenyan Society: USAID & the Restructuring of Health Care', *Review of African Political Economy* 25(75) (1998), pp. 89–100.
17. Videos are available at: http://heartsounds.ning.com, last accessed 2 February 2017.
18. *BRAIN GAIN: Training Peer Support Workers (PSWs) to Support Community Mental Health in Urban Uganda*, UKAID/DfID Medium Paired Institutional Partnership Progress Report, mPIP.14.
19. 'Butabika Plaintiffs Submissions' (Unpublished document, copy in possession of author).
20. Personal communication with Kabale Benon, 20 January 2018.

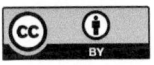

BIBLIOGRAPHY

UNPUBLISHED WORKS

Albert Cook Memorial Library, Makerere Medical School, Uganda (ACMM)

Mengo Hospital Case Notes.
Mengo Hospital Correspondence.
Medical Department Circular Memos.
Rwegellera, G. G. C., 'The Present State of Mental Health Services in Uganda and Proposals for Their Re-Organization, 1985–1986', Unpublished Paper.
Uganda Government, 'Ministry of Health Annual Report for the Year from 1st July 1963 to 30th June 1964', Typescript, 1964.

Bodleian Library, University of Oxford (BOD)

Micr.Afr.609(2), Papers of J. N. P. Davies.
Mss.Afr.s.1091, Papers of J. C. M. Baker.
Mss.Afr.s.1589, Papers of C. Baty.
Mss.Afr.s.1872(84), Papers of P. W. Hutton.
Mss.Afr.s.1872(144B), Papers of H. Trowell.
Mss.Afr.s.1872(153A-C). Papers of A. W. Williams.
Mss.Brit.Emp.S.22 G.552, Anti-Slavery Society Papers: Uganda.

© The Editor(s) (if applicable) and The Author(s) 2019
Y. Pringle, *Psychiatry and Decolonisation in Uganda*,
Mental Health in Historical Perspective,
https://doi.org/10.1057/978-1-137-60095-0

Jinja District Archives, Uganda (JDA)

Med 4/1, Psychiatric.

Kabale District Archives, Uganda (KDA)

Circulars.
JUD 1/3 I, Lunacy.
Minutes of the Kigezi District Team.

Mathari Hospital Records Project, Kenya

AF/M.132/55.

Mbale District Archives, Uganda (MDA)

MBL/4/57, Marriage, Customs, Witchcraft etc., 1943–1964.
MBL/4/68, Homicide in Bugisu.

Ministry of Health Archive, Uganda (UMOHA)

C90/ACR, Bosa Stephen B—Consult. Psychiat.
ECC.29, Consultants/Specialists—General.
First and Second Five-Year Development Plans—1961/66 and 1966/71.
GCH 9/2, Health Education.
GCT.8, Ministers' Tours (Excluding H.E. The President).
PH/ASC/42 (Box 56, Old Arrangement), Mental Health Advisory Committee: Association.
PH/ASC/46 (Box 29), Makerere Medical Graduates Association.
PHC/HP/2, Hospital—Butabika Hospital.
PH/HP/8 (Box 30 New), Butabika Hospital.

Ministry of Health Library, Uganda (UMOHL)

Raphael Owor, 'Report and Recommendations of the Health Policy Review Commission', Unpublished Report, 1987.

Mountains of the Moon University, Fort Portal, Uganda (MMU)

471(118), Loc Govt—Lunatics & Vagrants.
JUD 4(1), Lunacy.
MED 1079(295), Lunatics.

The National Archives, Kew, United Kingdom (TNA)

BW 90/16, East Africa—Medical School Mulago.
BW 90/190, Makerere University, Mulago Medical School and Hospital.
CO 536, Colonial Office: Uganda Original Correspondence.
CO 822, Colonial Office: East Africa: Original Correspondence.

Soroti District Archives, Uganda (SDA)

JUD 1/2, Lunatics.

Uganda National Archives (UNA)

A46/1120, Hoima Prison: Leper and Lunatic Prisoners.
C0524, Miscellaneous—Lunatics, Death of, in Kampala Jail.
C1266, Medical: Organisation of Medical Units at Kampala.
C1304, Benjamin Kagwa.
D107/12, Lunatics: Transport of Mental Patients.
J1/23, Medical Headquarters—Transfer of, to Kampala.
J142, Mental Hospital: Occupational Therapy for the Treatment of Patients.

World Health Organization Archives, Geneva (WHOA)

M-PROJECTS TANZANIA-30, Laughing Syndrome in Bukoba District.
M-PROJECTS UGANDA-38, Assistance to the Department of Psychiatry, Makerere University College.
M-PROJECTS UGANDA HMD-001, Faculty of Medicine, Makerere University, Uganda.
M4/86/12(B) Jkt 1, International Congresses of the World Federation of Mental Health.
M4/86/25(4), Fourth Pan African Psychiatric Congress, Abidjan, Ivory Coast, 30 June–5 July 1975.
M4/348/1 Jkt 1, General Information Re: Relations with Mental Health Organisations.
M4-372-28, Collaboration Between WHO & IPSER Regarding the International Programme on the Psychosocial Consequences of War Among Refugees & Displaced Persons.
M4/445/13, Carother's Study on Mental Health in Africans.
NIE-HMD-002 Jkt 1, Medical School, University of Ibadan.

World Health Organization Library, Geneva (WHOL)

AFR/MH/12, 'Training in Mental Health for Primary Health Care Workers', 1982.

OMH/74.3, Moser, J., 'Development of Mental Health Services in Africa', 1974.

OMH/EC/74.3, Moser, J., 'Approaches to the Development of Basic Mental Health Services', 1974, Paper Presented to the Expert Committee on Organization of Mental Health Services in Developing Countries, Geneva, 22–28 October 1974.

OMH/EC/74.7, Binitie, A., 'Mental Health Services in Developing Countries with Special Reference to Africa', 1974, Paper Presented to the Expert Committee on Organization of Mental Health Services in Developing Countries, Geneva, 22–28 October 1974.

OMH/EC/74.11, Sartorius, N., 'Immediate Needs in Mental Health Services: A Note for Discussion', 22 October 1974, Paper Presented to the Expert Committee on Organization of Mental Health Services in Developing Countries, Geneva, 22–28 October 1974.

MNH/POL/87.3, *African Mental Health Action Group, Tenth Meeting, Geneva, 8 May 1987.*

MNH/POL/88.2, Mental Health Leadership Training Workshop, Arusha, Tanzania, 3–14 August 1987.

NAD/UNHCR/WHO/RHB.9, *Equal Opportunities for All: A Community-Based Rehabilitation Project for Refugees, Kampala, Uganda, 23–27 September 1996.*

SEA/ME/Meet.Dir.Sch.P.H.4/23, Makerere University Medical School Country Report—Uganda, East Africa.

SEA/Ment./19 Annex 7, Recommendations of the International Workshop on Priorities in Mental Health Care (Held in Madurai, from 21 to 22 January 1971, Under the Auspices of the World Federation for Mental Health), n.d.

Theses

Baingana, F., 'Use Made of Ward 16 Old Mulago and Butabika Hospital: Patients Views About the Traditional Healer' (Unpublished MMed dissertation, Makerere University, 1987).

Beuschel, G. C., 'Shutting Africans Away: Lunacy, Race and Social Order in Colonial Kenya, 1910–1963' (Unpublished PhD thesis, University of London, 2001).

Billington, W. R., 'Neurosyphilis in Natives of East Africa' (Unpublished MD thesis, University of Cambridge, 1945).

Bracken, P. J., 'Trauma and the Age of Postmodernity: A Hermeneutic Approach to Post Traumatic Anxiety' (Unpublished PhD thesis, University of Warwick, 1998).

Earle, J. L., 'Political Theologies in Late Colonial Buganda' (PhD thesis, University of Cambridge, 2012).

Hurn, J. D., 'The History of General Paralysis of the Insane in Britain, 1830 to 1950' (Unpublished PhD thesis, University of London, 1998).

Khanakwa, P., 'Masculinity and Nation: Struggles in the Practice of Male Circumcision Among the Bagisu of Eastern Uganda, 1900s to 1960s' (Unpublished PhD thesis, Northwestern University, 2011).

Mahone, S., 'The Psychology of the Tropics: Conceptions of Tropical Danger and Lunacy in British East Africa' (Unpublished DPhil thesis, University of Oxford, 2004).

Tuck, M. W., 'Syphilis, Sexuality, and Social Control: A History of Venereal Disease in Colonial Uganda' (Unpublished PhD thesis, Northwestern University, 1997).

Zeller, D., 'The Establishment of Western Medicine in Buganda' (Unpublished PhD thesis, Columbia University, 1971).

Interviews and Personal Communication

Interview with J. Atukunda, Kampala, 17 August 2016.

Interview with R. Mpango, Kampala, 30 August 2016.

Interview with R. Busingye, 30 August 2016.

Interview with A. Nsimbi, Kampala, August 2016.

Interview with J. Odoki, Kampala, August 2016.

Interview with E. Nkururungi, Kampala, September 2016.

Interview with R. Alambuya, Jinja, September 2016.

Interview with B. Kabale, Kampala, September 2016.

Interview with P. Nabuto, Mpigi District, 19 October 2011, MPG-04.

Interview with S. Ndyanabangi, Ministry of Health, Kampala, 3 May 2011, NDY-01.

Interview with V. Wankiiri in Kampala, Uganda, 29 August 2011, WAN-01.

Interview with two Ganda females, Butabika, 16 May 2011, BUT-01.

Interview with Ganda male, Butabika, 24 May 2011, BUT-03.

Interview with Ganda female, Butabika, 23 June 2011, BUT-04.

Interview with Ankole male, approximately 71 years old, Butinde Village, Kebisoni Sub-County, Rukungiri District, 5 July 2011, RUK-06.

Interview with female nurse, Rwakabengo, Rukungiri District, 5 July 2011, RUK-10.

Interview with Ganda male, approximately 92 years old, Kawuku, Kayunga District, 3 June 2011, KAY-03.

Interview with Gisu male, approximately 80 years old, Mbale District, 27 October 2011, MLE-01.

Interview with Gisu male, approximately 81 years old, Mbale District, 27 October 2011, MLE-02.

Interview with Gisu female, approximately 81 years old, Mbale District, 27 October 2011, MLE-03.

Interview with Gisu female, approximately 75 years old, Mbale District, 27 October 2011, MLE-04.

Interview with Gisu female, approximately 60 years old, Mbale District, 27 October 2011, MLE-05.

Interview with Gisu male, approximately 74 years old, Mbale District, 27 October 2011, MLE-06.

Interview with Gisu female, approximately 61 years old, Mbale District, 27 October 2011, MLE-07.

Interview with Gisu female, approximately 80 years old, Mbale District, 27 October 2011, MLE-08.

Interview with Gisu female, approximately 80 years old, Mbale District, 27 October 2011, MLE-09.

Interview with Gisu male, approximately 70 years old, Mbale District, 27 October 2011, MLE-10.

Interview with Gisu male, approximately 71 years old, Mbale District, 27 October 2011, MLE-11.

Interview with Gisu male, approximately 77 years old, Mbale District, 27 October 2011, MLE-12.

Interview with Gisu female, approximately 74 years old, Mbale District, 27 October 2011, MLE-13.

Interview with Gisu female, approximately 70 years old, Mbale District, 31 October 2011, MLE-15.

Interview with Gisu female, approximately 78 years old, Mbale District, 1 November 2011, MLE-16.

Interview with Gisu male, approximately 77 years old, Mbale District, 1 November 2011, MLE-18.

Personal communication with G. A. German, 29 January 2012.

Personal communication with J. F. Wood, 7 October 2011.

Personal communication with W. Acuda, 21 October 2011.

Personal communication with J. Orley, 25 September 2011.

Personal communication with J. Bossa, 6 July 2012.

Personal communication with Kabale Benon, 20 January 2018

Other Unpublished Material, in My Possession

Alambuya, R., 'Human Rights Violations Experienced by People with Psychosocial Disabilities', Keynote address presented at the Launch of the WHO Quality Rights Project and Tool Kit, New York, 28 June 2012.

'Butabika Plaintiffs Submissions'.

Davies, D. L., 'Report on the Teaching of Psychiatry at Makerere University College Department of Psychiatry', Unpublished Report, 1969.

'Department of Psychiatry Annual Report, 1966–1967', *Makerere University College Reports, 1966–1967*, Kampala, 1967.

'Department of Psychiatry Annual Report, 1968–1969', *Makerere University College Reports, 1968–1969*, Kampala, 1969.

Dunlop, D. W., 'Health Care Financing: Recent Experience in Africa', Conference Paper delivered at 'Health and Development in Africa', University of Bayreuth, Germany, 2–4 June 1982.

Fuad, J., 'Insanity and the Law', Unpublished Seminar Paper, 1970.

Muhangi, J., 'Psychiatry in Kenya: New Horizons in Medical Care', Inaugural Lecture delivered at the University of Nairobi, 31 January 1980.

Wood, J. F., 'An Introduction to the Uganda Psychiatric Service', Unpublished Lecture, 1969.

Wood, J. F., 'Brain Syndromes (or Organic Confusional States)', Unpublished Lecture, 1969.

Wood, J. F., 'Psychiatry for Lawyers', Unpublished Lecture, 1970.

Wood, J. F., 'Rehabilitation & Psychiatry', Unpublished Lecture, n. d.

Websites

British Broadcasting Corporation, 'Physical Mental Health Treatments 1957, Part 1', last accessed 12 December 2012, at http://www.youtube.com/watch?v=2KxU3dPeink.

Heartsounds Website, last accessed 2 February 2017, at http://heartsounds.ning.com.

PUBLISHED WORKS

Newspapers

Daily Monitor
Ddoboozi lya Buganda
Gambuze
The Independent
Matalisi
New Vision
The Times
Uganda Argus
Uganda Herald

Reports and Official Publications

BRAIN GAIN: Training Peer Support Workers (PSWs) to Support Community Mental Health in Urban Uganda, UKAID/DfID Medium Paired Institutional Partnership Progress Report, mPIP.14.

'Declaration of Alma-Ata International Conference on Primary Health Care, Alma-Ata, USSR, 6–12 September 1978', http://www.who.int/publications/almaata_declaration_en.pdf, last accessed 23 February 2015.

Mental Disorders and Mental Health in Africa South of the Sahara: CCTA/CSA-WFMH-WHO Meeting of Specialists on Mental Health (Bukavu, 1958).

Mental Health Services in the Developing World: Reports on Workshops on Mental Health, Edinburgh (1968) and Kampala (1969), Commonwealth Foundation Occasional Paper, IV (Hove, 1969).

Proceedings of a Workshop on Alcohol and Drug Dependence of the Association of Psychiatrists in Africa (Nairobi, 1974).

Royal College of Psychiatrists, *Report of the Working Party to Review Psychiatric Practices and Training in a Multi-Ethnic Society*, Council Report CR48 (London, 1996).

The Report of the Commission of Inquiry into Violations of Human Rights: Verbatim Record of Proceedings, Vol. 1 (Kampala, 1994).

The Report of the Commission of Inquiry into Violations of Human Rights: Verbatim Record of Proceedings, Vol. 4 (Kampala 1994).

Uganda Constitutional Petition no. 64 of 2011.

Uganda Hansard, 99, Fourth Session (1970/71).

Uganda Government, *The First Five-Year Development Plan* (Entebbe, 1962).

Uganda Government, *The Mental Treatment Act, Chapter 270, Revised Edition*, 1964.

Uganda Medical and Dental Practitioners Council, Specialist Register. Available at: http://www.umdpc.com/registers/Specialist%20Register.xls. Last accessed 17 December 2017.

Uganda Protectorate, *Annual Reports of the Medical Department* (series).

Uganda Protectorate, *Annual Report on the Treatment of Offenders for the Year Ended 31st December, 1954* (Entebbe, 1955).

Uganda Protectorate, *Blue Books* (series).

Uganda Protectorate, *The Penal Code Act*, CAP 302 (Entebbe, 1950).

World Health Organization, *Reports of the Expert Committee on Mental Health* (series).

World Health Organization, *WHO and Mental Health 1949–1961* (Geneva, 1962).

World Health Organization, *The Work of WHO 1970: Annual Report of the Director-General to the World Health Assembly and to the United Nations* (Geneva, 1971).

World Health Organization, *Report of the International Pilot Study of Schizophrenia* (Geneva, 1973).

World Health Organization, *Mental Health Care in Developing Countries: A Critical Appraisal of Research Findings: Report of a WHO Study Group* (Geneva, 1984).

World Health Organization, *The Introduction of a Mental Health Component into Primary Health Care* (Geneva, 1990).

World Health Organization, *Diagnostic and Management Guidelines for Mental Disorders in Primary Care: ICD-10 Chapter V Primary Care Version* (Göttingen, 1996).

World Health Organization, *Prevention of Violence: A Public Health Priority*, Forty-Ninth World Health Assembly Resolution (Geneva, 20 May 1996).

World Health Organization, *WHO ProMIND: Profiles on Mental Health in Development: Uganda* (Geneva, 2012).

Other Printed

Abbo, C., 'Profiles and Outcome of Traditional Healing Practices of Severe Mental Illnesses in Two Districts of Eastern Uganda', *Global Health Action* 4 (2011), pp. 1–15.

Abramowitz, S., and C. Panter-Brick, 'Bringing Life into Relief: Comparative Ethnographies of Humanitarian Practice', in S. Abramowitz and C. Panter-Brick, eds., *Medical Humanitarianism: Ethnographies of Practice* (Philadelphia, 2015).

Allen, T., 'Understanding Alice: Uganda's Holy Spirit Movement in Context', *Africa: Journal of the International African Institute* 61(3) (1991), pp. 370–399.

Allen, T., and K. Vlassenroot, eds., *The Lord's Resistance Army: Myth and Reality* (London, 2010).

Allman, J., 'Nuclear Imperialism and the Pan-African Struggle for Peace and Freedom: Ghana, 1959–1962', *Souls* 10(2) (2008), pp. 83–102.

Amrith, S. S., *Decolonizing International Health: India and Southeast Asia, 1930–65* (Basingstoke, 2006).

Anderson, D. M., 'Exit from Empire: Counter-Insurgency and Decolonization in Kenya, 1952–1963,' in T. Clack and R. Johnson, eds., *At the End of Military Intervention: Historical, Theoretical and Applied Solutions to Transition, Handover and Withdrawal* (Oxford, 2014).

Anderson, D. M., and R. Rathbone, 'Urban Africa: Histories in the Making', in D. M. Anderson and R. Rathbone, eds., *Africa's Urban Past* (Oxford, 2000).

Anderson, D. M., and Ø. H. Rolandsen, 'Violence as Politics in Eastern Africa, 1940–1990: Legacy, Agency, Contingency', *Journal of Eastern African Studies* 8(4) (2014), pp. 539–557.

Apter, D. E., *The Political Kingdom in Uganda: A Study of Bureaucratic Nationalism* (Princeton, NJ, 1967).

Arya, O. P., and F. J. Bennett, 'Venereal Disease in an Elite Group (University Students) in East Africa', *British Journal of Venereal Diseases* 43 (1967), pp. 275–279.

Assael, M. I., 'Changing Society and Mental Health in Eastern Africa', *Israel Annals of Psychiatry and Related Disciplines* 8 (1970), pp. 52–74.

Assael, M. I., J. M. Namboze, G. A. German, and F. J. Bennett, 'Psychiatric Disturbances During Pregnancy in a Rural Group of African Women', *Social Science & Medicine* 6(3) (1972), pp. 387–395.

Baasher, T. A., G. M. Carstairs, R. Giel, and F. R. Hassler, eds., *Mental Health Services in Developing Countries: Papers Presented at a WHO Seminar on the Organization of Mental Health Services, Addis Ababa, 27 November to 4 December 1973* (Geneva, 1975).

Baasher, T., A. S. E. D. Elhakim, K. El Fawal, and V. B. Wankiiri, 'On Vagrancy and Psychosis', *Community Mental Health Journal* 19(1) (1983), pp. 27–41.

Babumba, E. M., 'An African Patient', *East African Medical Journal* 31(8) (1954), pp. 373–376.

Baillie, D., M. Aligawesa, H. Birabwa-Oketcho, C. Hall, D. Kyaligonza, R. Mpango, M. Mulimira, and J. Boardman, 'Diaspora and Peer Support Working: Benefits of and Challenges for the Butabika-East London Link', *BJPsych International*, 12(1) (2015), pp. 10–13.

Bains, J., 'Race, Culture and Psychiatry: A History of Transcultural Psychiatry', *History of Psychiatry* 16 (2005), pp. 139–154.

Barnett, M. N., and M. Finnemore, 'The Politics, Power, and Pathologies of International Organizations', *International Organization* 53(4) (1999), pp. 699–732.

Bartholomew, R. E., 'Tarantism, Dancing Mania and Demonopathy: The Anthro-Political Aspects of "Mass Psychogenic Illness"', *Psychological Medicine* 24 (1994), pp. 281–307.

Bass, A. Z., 'Promoting Nationhood Through Television in Africa', *Journal of Broadcasting* 13(2) (1969), pp. 163–166.

Beck, A., *A History of the British Medical Administration of East Africa: 1900–1950* (Cambridge, MA, 1970).

Behrend, H., *Alice Lakwena and the Holy Spirits: War in Northern Uganda, 1985–97* (Ohio, 2000).

Bennett, F. J., 'Medical Manpower in East Africa: Prospects and Problems', *East African Medical Journal* 42(4) (1965), pp. 149–161.

Bennett, F. J., and M. I. Assael, 'The Mental Health of Immigrants and Refugees from Rwanda at Kasangati, Uganda', *Psychopathologie Africaine* 6(3) (1970), pp. 321–334.

Bennett, F. J., and A. Mugalula-Mukiibi, 'An Analysis of People Living Alone in a Rural Community in East Africa', *Social Science & Medicine* 1 (1967), pp. 97–115.

Bennett, F. J., and H. Senkatuka, 'Health Education Via Mass Media', *Journal of Tropical Pediatrics* 12(supp3) (1966), pp. 31–32.

Bennett, F. J., G. A. Saxton, and A. Mugalula-Mukiibi, 'Kasangati—The Background to a Health Centre', in F. J. Bennett, ed., *Nkanga: Special Edition on Medicine and Social Sciences in East and West Africa* (Kampala, 1973).

Bennett, F. J., G. A. Saxton, J. Namboze, and H. L. Matovu, 'Kasangati Health Centre 1959–1972', in F. J. Bennett, ed., *Nkanga: Special Edition on Medicine and Social Sciences in East and West Africa* (Kampala, 1973).

Bernard, V., 'Violence Against Health Care: Giving in Is Not an Option', *International Review of the Red Cross* 95(889) (2013), pp. 5–12.

Bernstein, B., 'Social Class, Speech Systems and Psycho-Therapy', *The British Journal of Sociology* 15(1) (1964), pp. 54–64.

Bevan, J., 'The Myth of Madness: Cold Rationality and 'Resource' Plunder by the Lord's Resistance Army', *Civil Wars* 9(4) (2007), pp. 343–358.

Bhugra, D., 'Professor John Cox', *Psychiatric Bulletin*, 27 (2003), p. 471.

Bibeau, G., and E. Corin, 'Dr. Ravi L. Kapur (1938–2006): A Psychiatrist at the Crossroads of Multiple Worlds', *Transcultural Psychiatry* 47 (2010), pp. 159–180.

Birn, A.-E., 'The Stages of International (Global) Health: Histories of Success or Successes of History?' *Global Public Health: An International Journal for Research, Policy and Practice* 4(1) (2009), pp. 50–68.

Boardman, J., and E. Ovuga, 'Rebuilding Psychiatry in Uganda', *Psychiatric Bulletin* 21(10) (1997), pp. 649–655.

Bracken, P. J., J. E. Giller, and S. Kabaganda, 'Helping Victims of Violence in Uganda', *Medicine and War* 8(3) (1992), pp. 155–163.

Bracken, P. J., J. E. Giller, and D. Summerfield, 'Psychological Responses to War and Atrocity: The Limitations of Current Concepts', *Social Science & Medicine* 40(8) (1995), pp. 1073–1082.

Bracken, P. J., J. E. Giller, and D. Summerfield, 'Rethinking Mental Health Work with Survivors of Wartime Violence and Refugees', *Journal of Refugee Studies* 10(4) (1997), pp. 431–442.

Branch, A., 'Humanitarianism, Violence, and the Camp in Northern Uganda', *Civil Wars* 11(4) (2009), pp. 477–501.

Branch, A., *Displacing Human Rights: War and Intervention in Northern Uganda* (Oxford, 2011).

Brazier, F. S., 'The Incident at Nyakishenyi, 1917', *Uganda Journal* 32(1) (1968), pp. 17–27.

Brett, A., 'Testimonies of War Trauma in Uganda', in Tim Allen, ed., *In Search of Cool Ground: War, Flight and Homecoming in Northeast Africa* (Laurenceville, 1996).

Bridges, R., and M. Posnansky, 'African History at Makerere in the 1960s: A Further Perspective', *History in Africa* 31 (2004), pp. 479–482.

Brody, E. B., 'The World Federation for Mental Health: Its Origins and Contemporary Relevance to WHO and WPA Policies', *World Psychiatry* 3(1) (2004), pp. 54–55.

Bullard, A., 'Imperial Networks and Postcolonial Independence: The Transition from Colonial to Transcultural Psychiatry', in S. Mahone and M. Vaughan, eds., *Psychiatry and Empire* (Basingstoke, 2007).

Burnham, J. C., 'Transnational History of Medicine After 1950: Framing and Interrogation from Psychiatric Journals', *Medical History* 55(1) (2011), pp. 3–26.

Burton, A., 'The Haven of Peace Purged: Tackling the Undesirable and Unproductive Poor in Dar es Salaam, *ca.* 1950s–1980s', *International Journal of African Historical Studies* 40(1) (2007), pp. 119–151.

Burton, A., and M. Jennings, 'Introduction: The Emperor's New Clothes? Continuities in Governance in Late Colonial and Early Postcolonial East Africa', *International Journal of African Historical Studies* 40(1) (2007), pp. 1–25.

Campbell, C., *Race and Empire: Eugenics in Colonial Kenya* (Manchester, 2007).

Carothers, J. C., 'A Study of Mental Derangement in Africans, and an Attempt to Explain Its Peculiarities, More Especially in Relation to the African Attitude to Life', *East African Medical Journal* 25(5) (1948), pp. 142–166.

Carothers, J. C., 'A Study of Mental Derangement in Africans, and an Attempt to Explain Its Peculiarities, More Especially in Relation to the African Attitude to Life', *East African Medical Journal* 25(5) (1948), pp. 197–219.

Carothers, J. C., *The African Mind in Health and Disease: A Study in Ethnopsychiatry* (Geneva, 1952).

Carothers, J. C., *The Psychology of Mau Mau* (Nairobi, 1955).

Carstairs, G. M., 'Psychiatric Problems of Developing Countries', *The British Journal of Psychiatry* 123(574) (1973), pp. 271–277.

Carstairs, G. M., and J. K. Wing, 'Attitudes of the General Public to Mental Illness', *British Medical Journal* (6 September 1958), pp. 594–597.

Carstairs, G. M., et al., 'Psychiatric Education: Survey of Undergraduate Psychiatric Teaching in the United Kingdom (1966–1967)', *British Journal of Psychiatry* 144 (1968), pp. 1411–1416.

Cheney, K., 'Locating Neocolonialism, "Tradition," and Human Rights in Uganda's "Gay Death Penalty"', *African Studies Review* 55(2) (2012), pp. 77–95.

Chorev, N., *The World Health Organization Between North and South* (Ithaca, 2012).

Conley, R., 'Laughing Malady Puzzle in Africa', *New York Times*, 8 August 1963, p. 29.

Cook, A. R., 'A Visit to a Branch Dispensary and a Sleeping Sickness Camp in Uganda', *Mercy and Truth* 148 (1909), pp. 105–109.

Cook, A. R., *Uganda Memories, 1897–1940* (Kampala, 1945).

Cooper, F., *Africa Since 1940: The Past of the Present* (Cambridge, 2002).

Cooper, S., 'Global Mental Health and Its Critics: Moving Beyond the Impasse', *Critical Public Health* 26(4) (2016), pp. 355–358.

Cooper, F., and A. L. Stoler, *Tensions of Empire: Colonial Cultures in a Bourgeois World* (Berkeley and Los Angeles, 1997).

Corin, E., and H. B. M. Murphy, 'Psychiatric Perspectives in Africa Part I: The Western Viewpoint', *Transcultural Psychiatry* 16(2) (1979), pp. 147–178.

Cox, J. L., 'Psychiatric Morbidity and Childbirth: A Prospective Study from Kasangati Health Centre, Kampala', *Proceedings of the Royal Society of Medicine* 69(3) (1976), pp. 221–222.

Cox, J. L., 'Aspects of Transcultural Psychiatry', *The British Journal of Psychiatry* 130(3) (1977), pp. 211–221.

Cox, J. L., 'Amakiro: A Ugandan Puerperal Psychosis?' *Social Psychiatry* 14(1) (1979), pp. 49–52.

Cox, J. L., 'Cultural Psychiatry, Diversity and Political Correctness in a Shrinking World', *International Psychiatry* 5(2) (2008), pp. 27–28.

Crammer, J. L., 'Training and Education in British Psychiatry 1770–1970', in H. Freeman and G. Berrios, eds., *150 Years of British Psychiatry* (London, 1996).

Crozier, A., *Practising Colonial Medicine: The Colonial Medical Service in British East Africa* (London, 2007).

Cueto, M., 'The Origins of Primary Health Care and Selective Primary Health Care', *American Journal of Public Health* 94(11) (2004), pp. 1864–1874.

Dahlberg, L. L., and J. A. Mercy, 'History of Violence as a Public Health Problem', *Virtual Mentor: American Medical Association Journal of Ethics* 11(2) (2009), pp. 167–172.

Davidson, A., 'Choreomania: An Historical Sketch, with Some Account of an Epidemic Observed in Madagascar', *Edinburgh Medical Journal* XIII (1867), pp. 124–136.

Davidson, R., 'Psychiatry and Homosexuality in Mid-Twentieth-Century Edinburgh: The View from Jordanburn Nerve Hospital', *History of Psychiatry* 20(4) (2009), pp. 403–424.

Davies, J. N. P., 'The History of the Uganda Branch of the British Medical Association, 1913 to 1932', *East African Medical Journal* 31(3) (1954), pp. 93–99.

de Jong, J. T. V. M., 'Prevention of the Consequences of Man-Made or Natural Disaster at the (Inter)National, the Community, the Family and the

Individual Level', in S. E. Hobfoll and M. W. de Vries, eds., *Extreme Stress and Communities: Impact and Intervention* (Dordrecht, 1995).

Dick, G. W. A., 'A Preliminary Evaluation of the Immunizing Power of Chick-Embryo 17D Yellow Fever Vaccine Inoculated by Scarification', *American Journal of Epidemiology* 55(1) (1952), pp. 140–153.

Dick, G. W. A., and E. S. Horgan, 'Vaccination by Scarification with a Combined 17D Yellow Fever and Vaccinia Vaccine', *The Journal of Hygiene* 50(3) (1952), pp. 376–383.

Dinwiddy, H., 'The Ugandan Army and Makerere Under Obote, 1962–71', *African Affairs* 82(326) (1983), pp. 43–59.

Diop, S. M. B., *The Place of Mental Health in the Development of Public Health Services*, AFRO Technical Papers no. 8 (Brazzaville, 1974).

Dodge, C. P., and P. D. Wiebe, eds., *Crisis in Uganda: The Breakdown of Health Services* (Oxford, 1985).

Dodge, C. P., and M. Raundalen, *Reaching Children in War: Sudan, Uganda and Mozambique* (Bergen, 1991).

Doom, R., and K. Vlassenroot, 'Kony's Message: A New *Koine?* The Lord's Resistance Army in Northern Uganda', *African Affairs* 98(390) (1999), pp. 5–36.

Dunbar, A. R., *A History of Bunyoro-Kitara* (Nairobi, 1965).

Dyregrov, A., and M. Raundalen, 'Children and the Stresses of War—A Review', in C. P. Dodge and M. Raundalen, eds., *War, Violence and Children in Uganda* (Oslo, 1987).

Earle, J. L., 'Reading Revolution in Late Colonial Buganda', *Journal of Eastern African Studies* 6(3) (2012), pp. 507–526.

Ebrahim, G. J., 'Mass Hysteria in School Children: Notes on Three Outbreaks in East Africa', *Afya* 3(10) (1969), pp. 7–9.

'Editorial', *East African Medical Journal* 25(1) (1948), p. 1.

Egdell, H. G., 'A Rural Psychiatric Service in Uganda', *Psychopathologie Africaine* 6(1) (1970), pp. 87–94.

Egdell, H. G., 'The Medical Assistant and Psychiatric Care', *Psychopathologie Africaine* 6(1) (1970), pp. 83–86.

Egdell, H. G., 'Obituary of Steven Bosa', *The Psychiatrist* 25 (2001).

Egdell, H. G., and J. P. Stanfield, 'Paediatric Neurology in Africa: A Ugandan Report', *British Medical Journal* (February 1972), pp. 548–552.

'Epidemic Hysteria', *British Medical Journal* (November 1966), p. 1280.

Ernst, W., *Mad Tales from the Raj: Colonial Psychiatry in South Asia, 1800–58* (London, 2010).

Ernst, W., *Colonialism and Transnational Psychiatry: The Development of an Indian Mental Hospital in British India, c. 1925–1940* (London, 2013).

Ernst, W., and T. Mueller, eds., *Transnational Psychiatries: Social and Cultural Histories of Psychiatry in Comparative Perspective c. 1800–2000* (Newcastle, 2010).

Fanon, F., *The Wretched of the Earth*, trans. R. Philcox (New York, 1963).

Fassin, D., and R. Rechtman, *The Empire of Trauma: An Inquiry into the Condition of Victimhood* (Princeton, 2009).

Feierman, S., 'Change in African Therapeutic Systems', *Social Science and Medicine* 13B (1979), pp. 227–284.

Feierman, S., 'Colonizers, Scholars, and the Creation of Invisible Histories', in V. E. Bonnell and L. Hunt, eds., *Beyond the Cultural Turn: New Directions in the Study of Society and Culture* (Berkeley and Los Angeles, 1999).

Foster, W. D., *The Early History of Scientific Medicine in Uganda* (Nairobi, 1970).

Foster, W. D., 'Makerere Medical School: 50th Anniversary', *British Medical Journal* 3(5932) (1974), p. 675.

German, G. A., 'The Psychiatry of Poverty', *Psychopathologie Africaine* 7(1) (1971), pp. 113–117.

German, G. A., 'Aspects of Clinical Psychiatry in Sub-Saharan Africa', *The British Journal of Psychiatry* 121(564) (1972), pp. 461–479.

German, G. A., and O. P. Arya, 'Psychiatric Morbidity Amongst a Uganda Student Population', *British Journal of Psychiatry* 115 (1969), pp. 1323–1329.

German, G. A., and M. I. Assael, 'Achievement Stress and Psychiatric Disorders Amongst Students in Uganda', *Israel Annals of Psychiatry and Related Disciplines* 9(1) (1971), pp. 30–38.

German, G. A., and A. C. Raman, 'From Birth to Maturity—Historical Aspects of the Association of Psychiatrists in Africa', *African Journal of Psychiatry* 2(2) (1976), pp. 255–265.

Giel, R., and T. W. Harding, 'Psychiatric Priorities in Developing Countries', *British Journal of Psychiatry* 128(6) (1976), pp. 513–522.

Gijswijt-Hofstra, M., and H. Oosterhuis, 'Introduction: Comparing National Cultures of Psychiatry', in M. Gijswijt-Hofstra, H. Oosterhuis, J. Vijselaar, and H. Freeman, eds., *Psychiatric Cultures Compared: Psychiatry and Mental Health Care in the Twentieth Century: Comparisons and Approaches* (Amsterdam, 2005).

Gijswijt-Hofstra, M., H. Oosterhuis, J. Vijselaar, and H. Freeman, eds., *Psychiatric Cultures Compared: Psychiatry and Mental Health Care in the Twentieth Century: Comparisons and Approaches* (Amsterdam, 2005).

Giller, J., 'Caring for "Victims of Torture" in Uganda: Some Personal Reflections', in P. J. Bracken and C. Petty, eds., *Rethinking the Trauma of War* (London, 1998).

Gish, O., 'Selective Primary Care: Old Wine in New Bottles', *Social Science and Medicine* 16(10) (1982), pp. 1049–1054.

Githiora, B., 'The African Centre for the Treatment and Rehabilitation of Torture Victims: Treating the Terrified', *Executive*, December 1993, pp. 43–44.

Goldthorpe, J. E., *An African Elite: Makerere College Students 1922–1960* (Nairobi, 1965).

Graboyes, M., 'Chappati Complaints and Biriani Cravings: The Aesthetics of Food in Colonial Zanzibari Institutions', *Journal of Eastern African Studies* 5(2) (2011), pp. 313–328.

Graboyes, M., *The Experiment Must Continue: Medical Research and Ethics in East Africa, 1940–2014* (Athens, OH, 2015).

Green, A., 'Margaret Mungherera', *The Lancet* 389 (March 2017), p. 1188.

Grob, G. N., 'The Attack of Psychiatric Legitimacy in the 1960s: Rhetoric and Reality', *Journal of the History of the Behavioral Sciences* 47(4) (2011), pp. 398–416.

Gureje, O., and A. Alem, 'Hidden Science? A Glimpse at Some Work in Africa', *World Psychiatry* 3(3) (2004), pp. 178–181.

Gureje, O., et al., 'Results from the Ibadan Centre', in T. B. Üstün and N. Sartorius, eds., *Mental Illness in General Health Care: An International Study* (Chichester, 1995).

Hall, J., 'Some Aspects of Economic Development in Uganda', *African Affairs* 51(203) (1952), pp. 124–134.

Hansen, H. B., 'The Colonial Control of Spirit Cults in Uganda', in D. M. Anderson and D. H. Johnson, eds., *Revealing Prophets: Prophecy in Eastern African History* (London, 1995).

Hansen, H. B., 'Uganda in the 1970s: A Decade of Paradoxes and Ambiguities', *Journal of Eastern African Studies* 7(1) (2013), pp. 83–103.

Harding, T. W., 'Introduction: Mental Health Services in the Developing Countries: The Issues Involved', in T. A. Baasher, G. M. Carstairs, R. Giel, and F. R. Hassler, eds., *Mental Health Services in Developing Countries: Papers Presented at a WHO Seminar on the Organization of Mental Health Services, Addis Ababa, 27 November to 4 December 1973* (Geneva, 1975).

Harrell-Bond, B. E., *Imposing Aid: Emergency Assistance to Refugees* (Oxford, 1986).

Harrell-Bond, B., 'Foreword', in F. L. Ahearn, ed., *Psychosocial Wellness of Refugees: Issues in Qualitative and Quantitative Research* (New York, 2000).

Harris, F. J., *Social Casework: An Introduction for Students in Developing Countries* (Nairobi, 1970).

Haskell, D., 'Educational Television in Uganda', *Today's Speech* 19(4) (1971), pp. 43–49.

Haynes, D. M., 'Framing Tropical Disease in London: Patrick Manson, *Filaria Perstans*, and the Uganda Sleeping Sickness Epidemic, 1891–1902', *Social History of Medicine* 13(3) (2000), pp. 467–493.

Heald, S., 'Mafias in Africa: The Rise of Drinking Companies and Vigilante Groups in Bugisu District, Uganda', *Africa* 56 (1986), pp. 446–467.

Heald, S., *Controlling Anger: The Anthropology of Gisu Violence* (Oxford, 1998).

Hearn, J., 'The "NGO-Isation" of Kenyan Society: USAID & the Restructuring of Health Care', *Review of African Political Economy* 25(75) (1998), pp. 89–100.

Heaton, M. M., *Black Skin, White Coats: Nigerian Psychiatrists, Decolonization, and the Globalization of Psychiatry* (Ohio, 2013).

Heinlein, F., *British Government Policy and Decolonisation 1945–1963: Scrutinising the Official Mind* (London, 2002).

Henckes, N., 'Narratives of Change and Reform Processes: Global and Local Transactions in French Psychiatric Hospital Reform After the Second World War', *Social Science & Medicine* 68(3) (2009), pp. 511–518.

Herskovits, M. J., '*The African Mind in Health and Disease: A Study in Ethnopsychiatry* by J. C. Carothers', *Man* 54 (1954), pp. 30–31.

Hoad, N., *African Intimacies: Race, Homosexuality, and Globalization* (Minneapolis, 2007).

Hooper, E., and L. Pirouet, *Uganda*, The Minority Rights Group Report No. 66 (London, 1989).

Hopkins, E., 'The Nyabingi Cult of Southwestern Uganda', in R. I. Rotberg and A. A. Mazrui, eds., *Protest and Power in Black Africa* (New York, 1970).

Hoppe, K. A., *Lords of the Fly: Sleeping Sickness Control in British East Africa, 1900–1960* (Westport, CN, 2003).

Hundle, A. K., 'Exceptions to the Expulsion: Violence, Security and Community Among Ugandan Asians, 1972–79', *Journal of Eastern African Studies* 7(1) (2013), pp. 164–182.

Iliffe, J., *East African Doctors: A History of the Modern Profession* (Kampala, 2002).

Jackson, L., *Surfacing Up: Psychiatry and Social Order in Colonial Zimbabwe, 1908–1968* (Ithaca & London, 2005).

Janzen, J., *The Quest for Therapy: Medical Pluralism in Lower Zaire* (Berkeley, 1978).

Jeffreys, M. D. W., 'Psychical Phenomena Among Negroes', *Journal of the Royal African Society* (1940), pp. 354–360.

Jilek, W. G., 'Emil Kraepelin and Comparative Sociocultural Psychiatry', *European Archives of Psychiatry and Clinical Neuroscience* 245(4–5) (1995), pp. 231–238.

Jilek-Aall, L., and W. G. Jilek, 'Culture and Mental Illness: A Study from Uganda by John H. Orley', *Transcultural Psychiatric Research Review* 10(2) (1973), pp. 149–152.

Jones, T. F., *Psychiatry, Mental Institutions, and the Mad in Apartheid South Africa* (Abingdon, 2012).

Jørgensen, J. J., *Uganda: A Modern History* (London, 1981).

Kagwa, B. H., 'The Problem of Mass Hysteria in East Africa', *East African Medical Journal* 41 (1964), pp. 560–566.

Kagwa, B. H., 'Observations on the Prevalence and Types of Mental Diseases in East Africa', *East African Medical Journal* 42 (1965), pp. 673–682.

Kagwa, B. H., 'Endemic Viral Encephalitis in Uganda', *East African Medical Journal* 44(8) (1967), pp. 333–342.

Kagwa, B. H., *A Ugandan: Defiant and Triumphant* (Hicksville, 1978).

Kapila, S., 'The "Godless" Freud and His Indian Friends: An Indian Agenda for Psychoanalysis', in S. Mahone and M. Vaughan, eds., *Psychiatry and Empire* (Basingstoke, 2007).

Kariara, J., 'The Dream of Africa', in D. Cook, ed., *Origin East Africa: A Makerere Anthology* (London, 1965).

Karugire, S. R., *A Political History of Uganda* (Kampala, 2010).

Kasozi, A. B. K., *The Social Origins of Violence in Uganda, 1964–1985* (Montreal, 1994).

Kavuma, P., *Crisis in Buganda, 1953–55: The Story of the Exile and Return of the Kabaka, Mutesa II* (London, 1979).

Keatley, P., 'Obituary: Idi Amin', *The Guardian*, 18 August 2003.

Keller, R. C., *Colonial Madness: Psychiatry in French North Africa* (Chicago, 2007).

Kibuka-Musoke, J., 'Amin's Madness by His Doctor: Exclusive', *The Observer*, 1 May 1977, p. 11.

Kigozi, F., and J. Ssebunnya, 'Integration of Mental Health into Primary Health Care in Uganda: Opportunities and Challenges', *Mental Health in Family Medicine* 6 (2009), pp. 37–42.

Kigozi, F., J. Ssebunnya, D. Kizza, S. Cooper, and S. Ndyanabangi, 'An Overview of Uganda's Mental Health Care System: Results from an Assessment Using the World Health Organization's Assessment Instrument for Mental Health Systems (WHO-AIMS)', *International Journal of Mental Health Systems* 4(1) (2010), pp. 1–9.

Kilroy-Marac, K., 'Of Shifting Economies and Making Ends Meet: The Changing Role of the Accompagnant at the Fann Psychiatric Clinic in Dakar, Senegal', *Culture, Medicine and Psychiatry* 38(3) (2014), pp. 427–447.

Kleinman, A. M., 'Depression, Somatization and the "New Cross-Cultural Psychiatry"', *Social Science & Medicine* 11(1) (1977), pp. 3–9.

Kodesh, N., 'Networks of Knowledge: Clanship and Collective Well-Being in Buganda', *The Journal of African History* 49(2) (2008), pp. 197–216.

Kodesh, N., *Beyond the Royal Gaze: Clanship and Public Healing in Buganda* (Charlottesville, 2010).

Kritsotaki, D., V. Long, and M. Smith, eds., *Deinstitutionalisation and After: Post-War Psychiatry in the Western World* (Basingstoke, 2016).

Kuhanen, J., *Poverty, Health and Reproduction in Early Colonial Uganda* (Joensuu, 2005).

La Fontaine, J., *The Gisu of Uganda* (London, 1959).

La Fontaine, J., 'Witchcraft in Bugisu', in J. Middleton and E. H. Winter, eds., *Witchcraft and Sorcery in East Africa* (London, 1963).

Lakoff, A., *Pharmaceutical Reason: Knowledge and Value in Global Psychiatry* (Cambridge, 2006).

Lambo, T. A., 'The Role of Cultural Factors in Paranoid Psychosis Among the Yoruba Tribe', *The British Journal of Psychiatry* 101(423) (1955), pp. 239–266.

Lambo, T. A., ed., *First Pan-African Psychiatric Conference Report* (Ibadan, 1961).

Lambo, T. A., 'Psychotherapy in Africa', *Psychotherapy and Psychosomatics* 24(4–6) (1974), pp. 311–326.

Lamwaka, C., 'Civil War and the Peace Process in Uganda, 1986–1997', *East African Journal of Peace and Human Rights* 4(2) (1998), pp. 139–169.

Lawn, J. E., J. Rohde, S. Rifkin, M. Were, V. K. Paul, and M. Chopra, 'Alma-Ata 30 Years On: Revolutionary, Relevant, and Time to Revitalise', *Lancet* 372(9642) (September 2008), pp. 917–927.

Laubscher, B. J. F., *Sex, Custom and Psychopathology: A Study of South African Pagan Natives* (London, 1937).

Leighton, A. H., et al., eds., *Psychiatric Disorders Among the Yoruba: A Report from the Cornell-Aro Mental Health Research Project in the Western Region, Nigeria* (Ithaca, NY, 1963).

Leon, C. A., 'Psychiatry in Latin America', *The British Journal of Psychiatry* 121(561) (1972), pp. 121–136.

Leopold, M., *Inside West Nile: Violence, History and Representation on an African Frontier* (Oxford, 2005).

Le Pape, M., and P. Salignon, eds., *Civilians Under Fire: Humanitarian Practices in the Congo Republic 1998–2000* (Brussels, 2003).

Lindblom, G., *The Akamba in British East Africa: An Ethnological Monograph* (Uppsala, 1920).

Lindfors, B., ed., *Africa Talks Back: Interviews with Anglophone African Authors* (Trenton, NJ, 2002).

Lindstrum, E., *Ruling Minds: Psychology in the British Empire* (Cambridge, MA, 2016).

Litsios, S., 'The Long and Difficult Road to Alma-Ata: A Personal Reflection', *International Journal of Health Services* 32(4) (2002), pp. 709–732.

Long, K., 'Rwanda's First Refugees: Tutsi Exile and International Response 1959–64', *Journal of Eastern African Studies* 6(2) (2012), pp. 211–229.

Loudon, J. B., 'Social Aspects of Ideas About Treatment', in A. V. S. de Reuck and R. Porter, eds., *Transcultural Psychiatry* (London, 1965).

Lyons, M., *The Colonial Disease: A Social History of Sleeping Sickness in Northern Zaire, 1900–1940* (Cambridge, 1992).

Lyons, M., 'The Power to Heal: African Medical Auxiliaries in Colonial Belgian Congo and Uganda', in D. Engels and S. Marks, eds., *Contesting Colonial Hegemony: State and Society in Africa and India* (London, 1994).

Lyons, M., 'Medicine and Morality: A Review of Responses to Sexually Transmitted Diseases in Uganda in the Twentieth Century', in P. W. Setel, M. Lewis, and M. Lyons, eds., *Histories of Sexually Transmitted Diseases and HIV/AIDS in Sub-Saharan Africa* (Westport, CT, 1999).

Mackay, D., 'A Background for African Psychiatry', *East African Medical Journal* 25(1) (1948), pp. 2–4.

Macpherson, M., 'Circumcision Year Names (Kamengilo) in Masaba & Their Meanings', *Uganda Journal* 39 (1980), pp. 59–75.

MacRae, J., A. B. Zwi, and L. Gilson, 'A Triple Burden for Health Sector Reform: "Post"-Conflict Rehabilitation in Uganda', *Social Science and Medicine* 42(7) (1996), pp. 1095–1108.

Mahone, S., 'The Psychology of Rebellion: Colonial Medical Responses to Dissent in British East Africa', *Journal of African History* 47(2) (2006), pp. 241–258.

Mahone, S., 'East African Psychiatry and the Practical Problems of Empire', in S. Mahone and M. Vaughan, eds., *Psychiatry and Empire* (Basingstoke, 2007).

Mahone, S., and M. Vaughan, eds., *Psychiatry and Empire* (Basingstoke, 2007).

Makerere College, *Report of the Council to the Assembly for the Year 1946* (Kampala, 1947).

Malkki, L. H., 'Speechless Emissaries: Refugees, Humanitarianism, and Dehistoricization', *Cultural Anthropology* 11(3) (1996), pp. 377–404.

'Manhattan Central Medical Society—N.Y.C.', *Journal of the National Medical Association* 41(1) (1949), p. 38.

Mayes, R., and A. V. Horwitz, 'DSM-III and the Revolution in the Classification of Mental Illness', *Journal of the History of the Behavioral Sciences* 41(3) (2005), pp. 249–267.

Mazrui, A. M., *Political Values and the Educated Class in Africa* (Berkeley and Los Angeles, 1978).

McCulloch, J., *Black Peril, White Virtue: Sexual Crime in Southern Rhodesia, 1902–1935* (Bloomington, IN, 2000)

McCulloch, J., *Colonial Psychiatry and 'the African Mind'* (Cambridge, 1995).

Miller, G., 'Is the Agenda for Global Mental Health a Form of Cultural Imperialism?' *Medical Humanities* (Published Online, 13 March 2014), pp. 1–4.

Mills, C., and S. Fernando, 'Globalising Mental Health or Pathologising the Global South? Mapping the Ethics, Theory and Practice of Global Mental Health', *Disability and the Global South* 1(2) (2014), pp. 188–202.

Mills, J., *Madness, Cannabis and Colonialism: The 'Native Only' Lunatic Asylums of British India, 1857 to 1900* (Basingstoke, 2000).

Mills, D., 'British Anthropology at the End of Empire: The Rise and Fall of the Colonial Social Science Research Council, 1944–1962', *Revue d'Histoire des Sciences Humaines* 6(1) (2002), pp. 161–188.

Moro, L. N., 'Interethnic Relations in Exile: The Politics of Ethnicity Among Sudanese Refugees in Uganda and Egypt', *Journal of Refugee Studies* 17(4) (2004), pp. 420–436.

Mulindwa, F., 'The *Bataka* Agitation and Resistance in Colonial Uganda', *Muwazo* 10(3) (2011), pp. 12–24.

Murray, T. W., 'Mental Health in Uganda', *Transcultural Psychiatric Research: Review and Newsletter* 1(1) (1964), p. 71.

Mutibwa, P., *The Buganda Factor in Uganda Politics* (Kampala, 2008).

Muwazi, E. M. K., and H. C. Trowell, 'Neurological Disease Among African Natives of Uganda', *East African Medical Journal* 21(1) (1944), pp. 2–19.

Nagenda, J., 'And This, At Last', in D. Cook, ed., *Origin East Africa: A Makerere Anthology* (London, 1965).

Neill, D., 'Paul Ehrlich's Colonial Connections: Scientific Networks and Sleeping Sickness Drug Therapy Research, 1900–1914', *Social History of Medicine* 22(1) (2008), pp. 61–77.

Neki, J. S., 'Psychiatry in South-East Asia', *The British Journal of Psychiatry* 123(574) (1973), pp. 257–269.

Nguyen, V.-K., *The Republic of Therapy: Triage and Sovereignty in West Africa's Time of AIDS* (Durham, 2010).

Noyes, A. P., and L. C. Kolb, *Modern Clinical Psychiatry*, 6th ed. (Philadelphia, 1963), pp. 430–436.

Nyombi, C., 'A Critical Review of the Uganda Mental Health Treatment Bill, 2011', *East African Journal of Peace and Human Rights* 18(2) (2012), pp. 499–513.

Odonga, A. M., *The First Fifty Years of Makerere Medical School and the Foundation of Scientific Medical Education in East Africa* (Kampala, 1989).

Organizacion Panamericana de la Salud, *Grupo de Trabajo Sobre La Administración de Servicios Psiquiátricos y de Salud Mental, Vina Del Mar, Chile, 14–19 de Abril de 1969* (Washington, DC, 1970).

Orley, J., *Culture and Mental Illness* (Nairobi, 1970).

Orley, J., 'A Prospective Study of 372 Consecutive Admissions to Butabika Hospital, Kampala', *East African Medical Journal* 49(1) (1972), pp. 16–26.

Orley, J., 'Indigenous Concepts of Disease and Their Interaction with Scientific Medicine', in E. E. Sabben-Clare, D. J. Bradley, and K. Kirkwood, eds., *Health in Tropical Africa During the Colonial Period: Based on the Proceedings of a Symposium Held at New College, Oxford, 21–23 March 1977* (Oxford, 1980).

Orley, J., 'Application of Promotion Principles', in *Preventing Mental Illness: Mental Health Promotion in Primary Care* (Chichester, 1998).

Orley, J. H., and J. P. Leff, 'The Effect of Psychiatric Education on Attitudes to Illness Among the Ganda', *The British Journal of Psychiatry* 121(2) (1972), pp. 137–141.

Orley, J., and J. K. Wing, 'Psychiatric Disorders in Two African Villages', *Archives of General Psychiatry* 36(5) (1979), pp. 513–520.

Ovuga, E., J. Boardman, and D. Wasserman, 'Integrating Mental Health into Primary Health Care: Local Initiatives from Uganda', *World Psychiatry* 6(1) (2007), pp. 60–61.

Parle, J., *States of Mind: Searching for Mental Health in Natal and Zululand, 1868–1918* (Scottsville, 2007).

Patel, V., and M. Prince, 'Global Mental Health: A New Global Health Field Comes of Age', *JAMA* 303(19) (2010), pp. 1976–1977.

Pearson-Patel, J., 'French Colonialism and the Battle Against the WHO Regional Office for Africa', *Hygiea Internationalis* 13(1) (2016), pp. 65–80.

Peterson, D. R., and E. C. Taylor, 'Rethinking the State in Idi Amin's Uganda: The Politics of Exhortation', *Journal of Eastern African Studies* 7(1) (2013), pp. 58–82.

Pols, H., 'Psychological Knowledge in a Colonial Context: Theories on the Nature of the "Native Mind" in the Former Dutch East Indies', *History of Psychology* 10(2) (2007), pp. 111–131.

Pressman, J. D., *Last Resort: Psychosurgery and the Limits of Medicine* (San Francisco, 1998).

Prince, R. H., 'The "Brain Fag" Syndrome in Nigerian Students', *Journal of Mental Science* 106 (1960), pp. 559–570.

Prince, R. H., 'What's in a Name?' *Transcultural Psychiatry* 34(1) (1997), pp. 151–154.

Pringle, Y., 'Crossing the Divide: Medical Missionaries and Government Service in Uganda, 1897–1940', in Anna Greenwood, ed., *Beyond the State: The Colonial Medical Services in British Africa* (Manchester, 2015).

Pringle, Y., 'Neurasthenia at Mengo Hospital, Uganda: A Case Study in Psychiatry and a Diagnosis, 1906–50', *The Journal of Imperial and Commonwealth History* 44(2) (2016), pp. 241–262.

Prunier, G., *Africa's World War: Congo, the Rwandan Genocide, and the Making of a Continental Catastrophe* (Oxford, 2009).

Rankin, A. M., and P. J. Philip, 'An Epidemic of Laughing in the Bukoba District of Tanganyika', *Central African Journal of Medicine* 9 (1963), pp. 167–170.

Raundalen, M., J. Lwanga, C. Mugisha, and A. Dyregrov, 'Four Investigations on Stress Among Children in Uganda', in C. P. Dodge and M. Raundalen, eds., *War, Violence and Children in Uganda* (Oslo, 1987).

Redfield, P., 'The Verge of Crisis: Doctors Without Borders in Uganda', in D. Fassin and M. Pandolfi, eds., *Contemporary States of Emergency: The Politics of Military and Humanitarian Interventions* (New York, 2010).

Reid, R., *A History of Modern Uganda* (Cambridge, 2017).

Roberts, G., 'The Uganda–Tanzania War, the Fall of Idi Amin, and the Failure of African Diplomacy, 1978–1979', *Journal of Eastern African Studies* 8(4) (2014), pp. 692–709.

Rosen, G., 'Psychopathology in the Social Process: I. A Study of the Persecution of Witches in Europe as a Contribution to the Understanding of Mass Delusions and Psychic Epidemics', *Journal of Health and Human Behaviour* 3 (1960), pp. 200–211.

Sadowsky, J., *Imperial Bedlam: Institutions of Madness in Colonial Southwest Nigeria* (Berkeley and Los Angeles, 1999).

Sartorius, N., 'Mental Health and Primary Health Care', *Mental Health in Family Medicine* 5 (2008), pp. 75–77.

Sartorius, N., and T. W. Harding, 'The WHO Collaborative Study on Strategies for Extending Mental Health Care, I: The Genesis of the Study', *American Journal of Psychiatry* 140 (1984), pp. 1470–1473.

Sembeguya, F. G., 'The Growth of an Indigenous Medical Profession', *East African Medical Journal* 41(2) (1964), pp. 39–45.

Sicherman, C., 'Ngugi's Colonial Education: "The Subversion...of the African Mind"', *African Studies Review* 38(3) (1995), pp. 11–41.

Sicherman, C., 'Building an African Department of History at Makerere, 1950–1972', *History in Africa* 30 (2003), pp. 253–282.

Sicherman, C., *Becoming an African University: Makerere, 1922–2000* (Trenton, 2005).

Siddiqi, J., *World Health and World Politics: The World Health Organization and the UN System* (London, 1995).

Simons, H. J., 'Mental Disease in Africans: Racial Determinism', *The British Journal of Psychiatry* 104(435) (April 1958), pp. 377–388.

Smartt, C. G. F., 'Mental Maladjustment in the East African', *British Journal of Mental Science* 102 (1956), 441–466.

Somnier, F. E., and I. K. Genefke, 'Psychotherapy for Victims of Torture', *The British Journal of Psychiatry* 149(3) (1986), pp. 323–329.

Southall, A. W., and P. C. W. Gutkind, *Townsmen in the Making: Kampala and Its Suburbs* (Kampala, 1957), pp. 149–150.

Ssekemwa, J. C., 'Witchcraft in Buganda Today', *Transition* 30 (1967), pp. 30–39.

Ssekamwa, J. C., *History and Development of Education in Uganda* (Kampala, 2000).

Sturdy, S., R. Freeman, and J. Smith-Merry, 'Making Knowledge for International Policy: WHO Europe and Mental Health Policy, 1970–2008', *Social History of Medicine* 26(3) (2013), pp. 532–554.

Summerfield, D., 'A Critique of Seven Assumptions Behind Psychological Trauma Programmes in War-Affected Areas', *Social Science & Medicine* 48(10) (1999), pp. 1449–1462.

Summerfield, D., 'Afterword: Against "Global Mental Health"', *Transcultural Psychiatry* 49(3–4) (2012), pp. 519–530.

Summers, C., 'Intimate Colonialism: The Imperial Production of Reproduction in Uganda, 1907–1925', *Signs* 16(4) (1991), pp. 787–807.

Summers, C., 'Grandfathers, Grandsons, Morality, and Radical Politics in Late Colonial Buganda', *International Journal of African Historical Studies* 38(5) (2005), pp. 427–447.

Summers, C., 'Radical Rudeness: Ugandan Social Critiques in the 1940s', *Journal of Social History* 39(3) (2006), pp. 741–770.

Summers, C., 'All the Kabaka's Wives: Marital Claims in Buganda's 1953–5 Kabaka Crisis', *The Journal of African History* 58(1) (2017), pp. 107–127.

Taithe, B., 'The Cradle of the New Humanitarian System? International Work and European Volunteers at the Cambodian Border Camps, 1979–1993', *Contemporary European History* 25(2) (2016), pp. 335–358.

Tamale, S., 'Out of the Closet: Unveiling Sexuality Discourses in Uganda', in C. M. Cole, T. Manuh, and S. F. Miescher, eds., *Africa After Gender?* (Bloomington, IN, 2007).

Taylor, F. K., and R. C. A. Hunter, 'Observation of a Hysterical Epidemic in a Hospital Ward', *Psychiatric Quarterly* 32 (1958), pp. 821–839.

Tewfik, G. I., 'A Hospital Visitors' Association', *The Lancet* (October 1956), p. 834.

Tewfik, G. I., 'Depression and E.C.T.', *East African Medical Journal* 34(4) (1957), pp. 137–142.

Tewfik, G. I., 'Mulago Hospital Clinical Staff Meeting 26 April 1958: The African Mind Fact or Myth?' *East African Medical Journal* 35(8) (1958), pp. 512–513.

Tewfik, G. I., 'Problems of Mental Illness in Uganda', *Mental Disorders and Mental Health in Africa South of the Sahara: CCTA/CSA-WFMH-WHO Meeting of Specialists on Mental Health* (Bukavu, 1958).

Tewfik, G. I., 'Psychoses in Africa', *Mental Disorders and Mental Health in Africa South of the Sahara: CCTA/CSA-WFMH-WHO Meeting of Specialists on Mental Health* (Bukavu, 1958).

Tewfik, G. I., 'Low Incidence of Fractures Among Africans Following Electro-Convulsive Therapy', *West African Medical Journal* 9(1) (1960), pp. 26–28.

Thompson, G., 'Colonialism in Crisis: The Uganda Disturbances of 1945', *African Affairs* 91 (1992), pp. 605–624.

Thomson, M., 'Mental Hygiene as an International Movement', in P. Weindling, ed., *International Health Organisations and Movements, 1918–1939* (Cambridge, 1995).

Ticktin, M., 'The Gendered Human of Humanitarianism: Medicalising and Politicising Sexual Violence', *Gender & History* 23(2) (2011), pp. 250–265.

Tripp, A. M., *Women and Politics in Uganda* (Oxford, 2000).

Trowell, H. C., 'Training Medical Practitioners', *East African Medical Journal* 33(7) (1956), pp. 253–258.

Vallely, P., 'I Genuinely Felt That by Being There I Could Moderate His Excesses', *The Times*, 10 December 1985, p. 5.

Vaughan, M., 'Idioms of Madness: Zomba Lunatic Asylum, Nyasaland, in the Colonial Period', *Journal of Southern African Studies* 9(2) (1983), pp. 218–238.

Vaughan, M., *Curing Their Ills: Colonial Power and African Illness* (Cambridge, 1991).

Vaughan, M., 'Changing the Subject? Psychological Counseling in Eastern Africa', *Public Culture* 28(3) 80 (2016), pp. 499–517.

Vokes, R., *Ghosts of Kanungu: Fertility, Secrecy & Exchange in the Great Lakes of East Africa* (Kampala, 2009).

Walugembe, J. E. (Post-humus), 'A Pioneer's Look at Psychotrauma in Uganda "Post-Traumatic Stress Disorder as Seen in Mulago Hospital Mental Health Clinic (1992)', *African Journal of Traumatic Stress* 1(1) (2010), pp. 6–18.

Wamboka, N. L., 'Uganda: Dr. Nakasi's Sacking Is Bad for Women in-Mates', *The Monitor*, 9 June 1998.

Wankiiri, V. B., 'Delivering Mental Health Through Primary Health Care: The Lesotho Experience', *Epidemiology and Community Psychiatry* (Boston, 1985).

Wankiiri, [V.] B., 'Problems in Achieving Mental Health for All in Southern Africa (Letter)', *World Health Forum* 12(2) (1991), pp. 210–211.

Watson, W. H., 'A Case of Sexual Perversion in an African Male', *East African Medical Journal* 20(10) (1943), p. 354.

Weindling, P., ed., *International Health Organisations and Movements, 1918–1939* (Cambridge, 1995).

Weisæth, L., 'Torture of a Norwegian Ship's Crew: The Torture, Stress Reactions and Psychiatric After-Effects', *Acta Psychiatrica Scandinavica* 80(s355) (1989), pp. 63–72.

White, L., *Speaking with Vampires: Rumor and History in Colonial Africa* (Berkeley, 2000).

Whitley, R., 'Global Mental Health: Concepts, Conflicts and Controversies', *Epidemiology and Psychiatric Sciences* 24(4) (2015), pp. 285–291.

Whyte, S. R., 'Penicillin, Battery Acid and Sacrifice', *Social Science and Medicine* 16 (1982), pp. 2055–2064.

Williams, A. W., 'The Next Generation', *East African Medical Journal* 34(10) (1957), pp. 521–528.

Wittkower, E. D., 'Transcultural Psychiatry', in J. G. Howells, ed., *Modern Perspectives in World Psychiatry* (Edinburgh, 1968).

Wood, J. F., 'A Half Century of Growth in Ugandan Psychiatry', *Uganda Atlas of Disease Distribution* (Kampala, 1968).

Wood, J. F., 'Utilising Therapeutic Potential in Psychiatric Hospital Staff', *Psychopathologie Africaine* 6(3) (1970), pp. 301–320.

Wrong, M., 'Mass Education in Africa', *African Affairs* (1944), pp. 105–111.

Wu, H. Y.-J., 'World Citizenship and the Emergence of the Social Psychiatry Project of the World Health Organization, 1948–c.1965', *History of Psychiatry* 26(2) (2015), pp. 166–181.

Wu, H. Y.-J., 'From Racialization to World Citizenship: The Transnationality of Taiwan and the Early Psychiatric Epidemiological Studies of the World Health Organization', *East Asian Science, Technology and Society* 10(2) (2016), pp. 183–205.

Youe, C. P., 'Peasants, Planters and Cotton Capitalists: The "Dual Economy" of Uganda', *Canadian Journal of African Studies* 12(2) (1978), pp. 163–184.

INDEX